Check out these video tutorials I made for the book! I hope this playlist will help you. Also, if you like, could you share how the book and videos worked for you? Thanks in advance!

Scan the QR code to watch the videos!

Do you have problem accessing the videos? Email me at avfitness99coaching@gmail.com and I'll sort it for you.

🎁 Join Our Community on Facebook for Exclusive Content!

Scan the QR Code Below 🎁

Disclaimer

wall pilates
workouts for women

Guess what? You get two cool gifts!

- A chart you can download.
  It helps you follow your exercises easily.

- A special way to text me if you have questions or just want to say hi!

Don't like texting? No problem! Email me anytime at **avfitness99coaching@gmail.com.**

I'm here to help you with your fitness!

Contents

CARDIO FOCUS

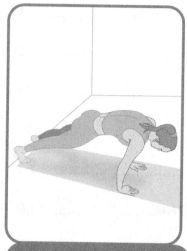

Dynamic Plank With Wall Support

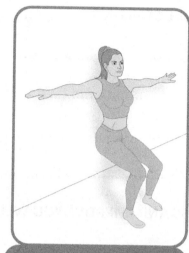

Wall Sit + Arm Circles

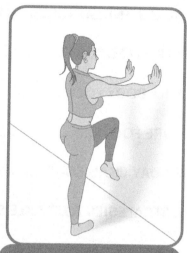

Wall Leg Raise + Kick Back

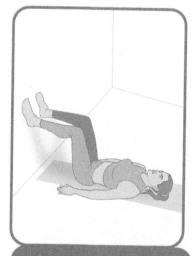

Wall Marches

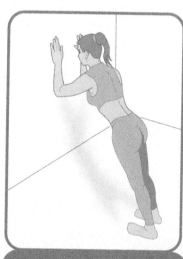

Wall Tricep Push-Up + Knee Raise

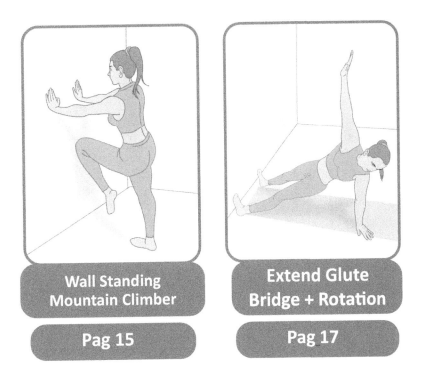

Wall Standing Mountain Climber

Extend Glute Bridge + Rotation

FULL BODY FOCUS

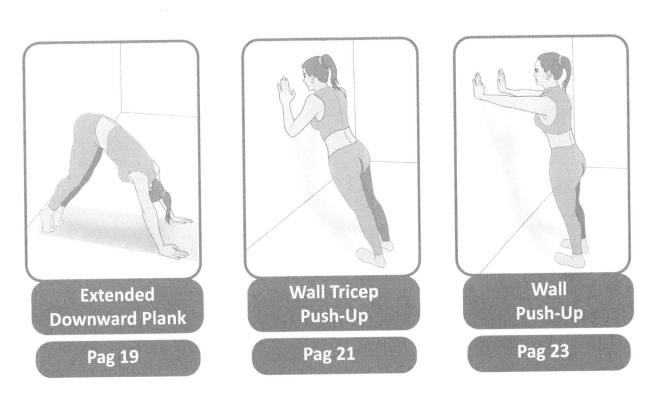

Extended Downward Plank

Wall Tricep Push-Up

Wall Push-Up

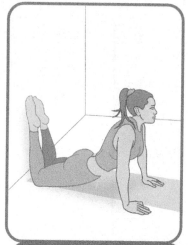

Kneeling Chest Raise

Pag 25

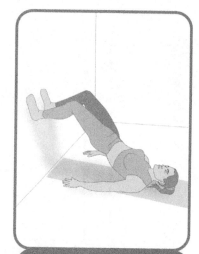

Wall Hip Thrust

Pag 27

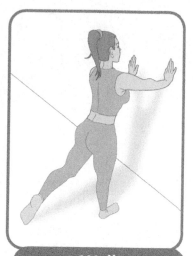

Wall Kick Back

Pag 29

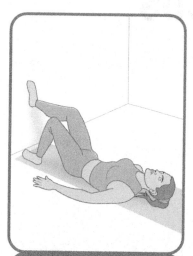

Wall Glute Bridge Half-Assisted

Pag 31

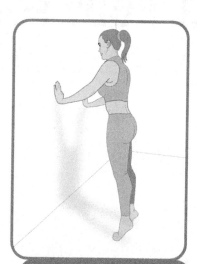

Wall Calf Raises

Pag 33

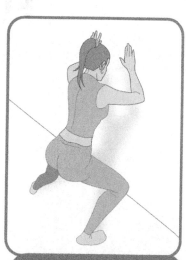

Wall Lateral Lunge

Pag 35

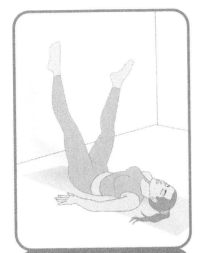

**Wall
Leg Lifts**

Pag 37

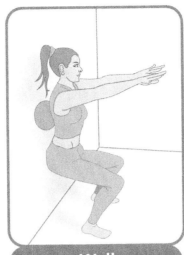

**Wall
Squats**

Pag 39

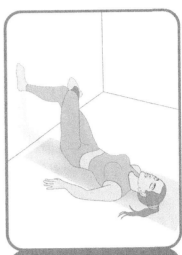

**Iso Leg Hold
Unilateral**

Pag 41

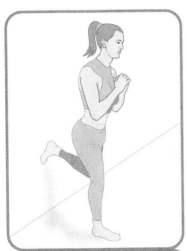

**Wall Split
Squat**

Pag 43

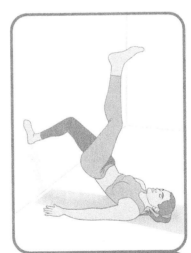

**Single Leg Wall
Glute Bridge**

Pag 45

CORE FOCUS

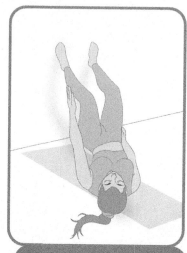

**Wall
Lateral Crunch**

Pag 47

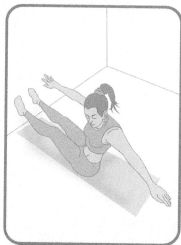

**Wall
Twist**

Pag 49

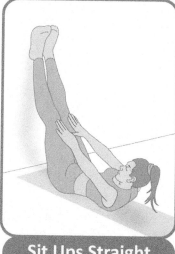

**Sit Ups Straight
Legged**

Pag 51

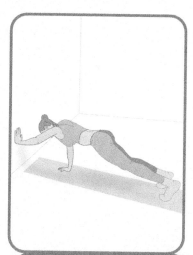

**Plank
Wall Touches**

Pag 53

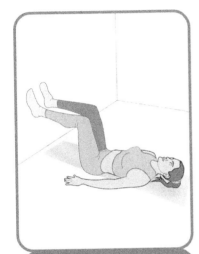

**Wall
Reverse Crunch**

Pag 55

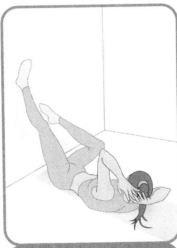

**Wall
Side Crunch**

Pag 57

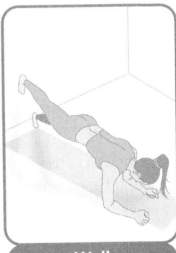

**Wall
Walking Plank**

Pag 59

WALL PILATES WORKOUTS

The 28-Day Body Sculpting Challenge to Tone your Abs and Glutes with Illustrated Full Body Routines.

Wall Pilates provides a full-body workout with a focus on the abdominal muscles, legs, and glutes.

Each exercise will not only strengthen your muscles but also help you relax your whole body through breathing tips. By training dozens of clients 1-on-1 with this methodology, I can assure you that the breathing cues present in each exercise make a huge difference in the effectiveness of the workout, giving you a sense of well-being and a boost of energy like no other type of exercise!

The Wall Pilates exercises selected in this book have been studied to provide benefits for women to burn calories, tone their abs, and improve their shapes. A wall is a great tool as it serves both as a resistance as well as support.

The workouts are suitable for both beginners and advanced as the exercises can be adjusted based on your fitness level, as suggested in the notes.

HOW YOUR BODY WILL CHANGE AFTER THESE WORKOUTS

As a Personal Trainer and having trained people 1-on-1 using wall Pilates exercises, I want to make sure that before starting working out you know exactly what you will get out of it.

I believe that "Wall Pilates Workout for Women" can really be a game-changer for your fitness level and give you the body (and also the mental health and peace of mind) you have been wanting for a long time.

Below are the main benefits you will obtain after performing these exercises (keep in mind that you will probably notice some changes in a few days, the people around you will notice it in two to three weeks, and after a month almost everyone you know will notice that something in you is changing!):

● **Muscle Toning**

There is a section called "Full Body Focus" that aims to strengthen and tone your whole body. This section has been studied specifically for women so that you will get your dream's body, having toned legs and an upper body slim (but still quite strong rather than skinny and weak).

Note: obviously, consistency is key to reach this goal.

● **More Flexibility and Balance**

By working on some unilateral exercises and working through a full range of motion, you will become more flexible, and your proprioception will increase. Training barefoot when doing wall Pilates is highly recommended. In many exercises you will be performing some reps with one side, and then switch to the other. This will make sure there are no imbalances in terms of balance, strength, and flexibility.

• Improved Posture

Through exercises that work your deep abdominal muscles, your posture will improve without the need to constantly think about how you sit or how you stand.It will simply become second nature to stand and sit with the perfect posture. I think that Wall Pilates is a great tool to counteract the effects of sitting for prolonged periods of time.

• More Relaxed

It will reduce your stress levels through daily exercises and breathing patterns that will enhance a sense of peace in your body. Moving daily will help you get rid of overthinking and anxiety that might impact your mental health. Also, during the exercises try to inhale through your nose, and exhale fully through your nose or mouth, with exhales always longer and deeper than inhalation. This is a key rule to make sure your body is relaxed, and you are in the present moment.

Imagine the benefits of focusing on a correct breathing pattern as well as doing effective exercises ...You will get close to a Superwoman!

• Improved Fitness

There will be some exercises daily that will aim to increase your heart rate and improve your cardiovascular health, making you fitter and feel better in just a few minutes per day. Towards the end of each workout there will be one to three exercises that will require you to move slightly faster and engage more muscles at the same time. This will make sure your heart rate goes up so that you will be burning more calories.

Let's see it this way: most of the exercise will make sure to tone your body making each muscle more defined. Then, by doing more "intense" exercises, you will get rid of some weight so that your shape will improve and be better than when you were in your early 20s!!

NOTES AND SUGGESTION BEFORE STARTING

1- It is important to execute the exercises as mentioned, with sets and reps to obtain maximal results. Failure to do so might compromise the results you want to achieve.

2- In the exercises where you will be asked to lay down, I suggest you use a mat because it might be uncomfortable laying down on the floor. Also, without a mat there is a possibility of slipping away from the wall, making the exercises less effective.

3- In the exercises that target your glutes (the ones in which you will lay down with your back), as already mentioned in the "how to do it" section as well as in the "note" section, it would be ideal to have your feet flat on the wall and knees bent at 90° aka having your thighs vertical to the floor. This will make sure that when you lift your hips and glutes, you will have maximal contraction. This will help toning your butt in no time!

What if you feel it too much on your hamstrings aka back of your thighs?

If you feel too much hamstrings involved, either come closer to the wall with your hips or lower down your feet a few inches. Another cue I like to give to my clients is to press with your heels on the wall. This will instantly work your glutes more.

4- If you don't have a wall available in your home (usually a corner is always found, but let's assume you don't have one at the moment), many people are also able to perform the following exercises using the backboard at the end of the bed in lying exercises and a door or closet for standing exercises.

The front door is another good solution as it is almost as firm as a wall.

5- Some people, albeit a very small percentage, show a lot of tiredness between the shoulder blades, as if all the fatigue is concentrated in that area of the body. If you should also have this feeling, do this: This is especially if they have not exercised in a while and now they started working out daily.

Firstly, if this is you, try to start exercising every second day rather than every day to let your body adapt to the new stimulus without overtraining it. Do this for a couple of weeks and then try start the challenge from zero once again.

CARDIO FOCUS

DYNAMIC PLANK WITH WALL SUPPORT

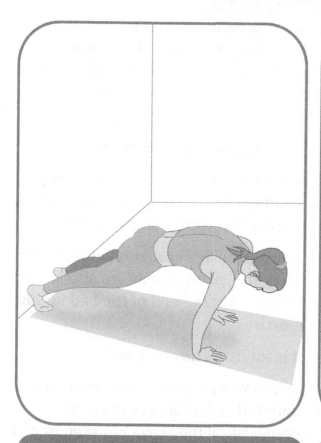

Step 1 - Plank position with arms straight and feet on the wall

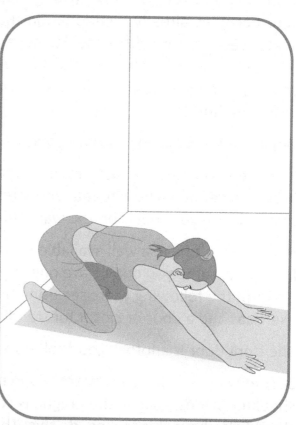

Step 2 - Bring your glutes towards the wall and stretch your back. Repeat for reps.

How to do it:

1. Set up in a plank position and place your feet against the wall (toes on the floor and soles of the feet on the wall). Keep your body and arms straight with hands below your shoulders.

2. Then, bring your glutes towards the wall by bending your knees. Keep your arms straight and feel a stretch on your back as you do so. Hold it for 1''.

3. Lastly, return into the starting position, and do it for the mentioned reps or for time.

Breathing:

As you go from plank position to moving your body close to the wall exhale fully. Then, inhale as you are coming back into the initial position.

Note:

Never let your knees touch the floor (or mat if you use one). The only contact point with the floor and wall are always feet and hands.

If you are a beginner, feel free to let your knees touch the floor. However, in a few sessions aim to do it "properly", without the knee assistance.

WALL SIT + ARM CIRCLES

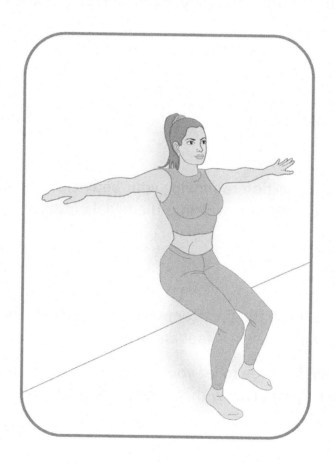

How to do it:

1. "Sit against the wall". Basically, place your back against the wall and bend your knees so that they are 90° with feet planted on the floor.

2. From this position, open your arms wide parallel to the floor and move them in small circles.

3. Keep doing it either for reps (counting circles you do), or time, as suggested in the workout routine.

Breathing:

No tips are needed, breath as normal. A tip that works with many people is to do a long exhale through the mouth. By doing that, they can hold the position for longer with less fatigue.

Note:

Great combo of exercise to work both your thighs as well as toning your arms and shoulders.

To make it slightly easier, feel free to "sit" a bit higher so that the angle of the knee is more than 90°, making the exercise more accessible for the first few sessions.

WALL LEG RAISE + KICK BACK

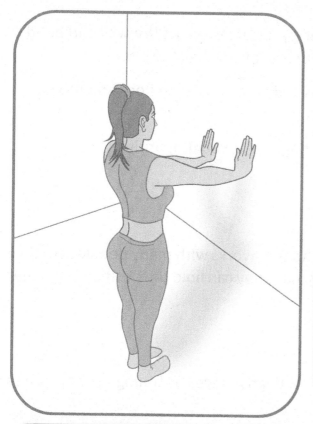

Step 1 - Starting position

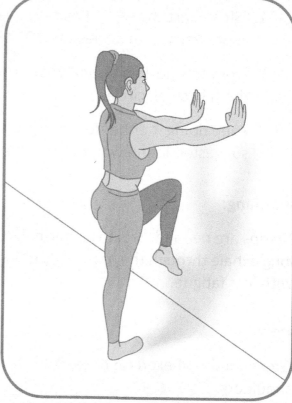

Step 2 - Lift one thigh parallel to the floor.

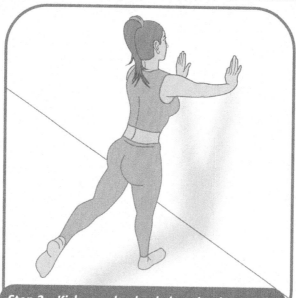

Step 3 – Kick your leg back, keeping it straight.
Repeat for reps, then switch sides.

How to do it:

1. Stand facing the wall an arm's distance from it. Keep feet slightly apart from each other and maintain your trunk straight.

2. Lift one thigh parallel to the floor whilst holding onto the wall with your hands for assistance. Hold it for 1''.

3. Then, kick the same leg back behind your body whilst keeping it straight. Hold 1'' contraction once you reach your full range of motion.

4. Keep repeating the sequence for the mentioned reps.

Breathing:

Breath as normal, no tips needed in this exercise. Avoid inhaling through your mouth if possible.

Note:

This is a great exercise because it works your balance, your hip flexor, glutes, and core strength as well as stretching the front of your thigh as you kick your leg back. The foot has to be in contact with the floor the whole time for maximal stability.

For an extra challenge, as you lift your thigh (let's say the left one, as shown in the image) parallel to the floor, also lift the heel of the opposite foot (so do a calf raise with the right foot). Then, once you kick your leg back, the planted foot comes back into its position. This would really test your balance and coordination.

WALL MARCHES

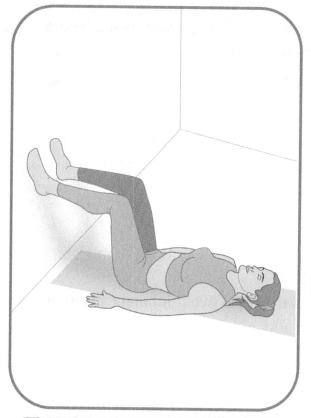

Step 1 – Set up.

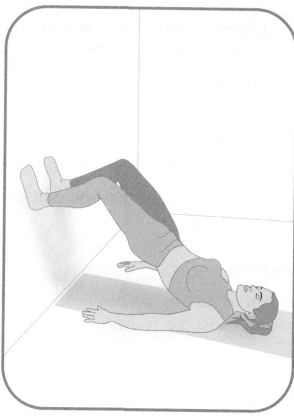

Step 2 – Starting position with hips lifted.

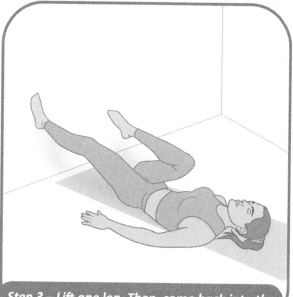

Step 3 – Lift one leg. Then, come back into the initial position and repeat with the other one.

How to do it:

1. Start with your back on the floor and your feet against the wall. Knees bent at 90° roughly (you can also put your feet higher than this). Arms on the side of your body resting on the floor.

2. From the set-up position, firstly lift your hips and contract your glutes. Keep this position whilst you lift one leg keeping your knee bent and move it towards your chest so that your thigh is vertical to the floor. Hold that position for a second.

3. Then, come back into the starting position, and do it on the other side. Keep going either for the mentioned seconds or for reps, as mentioned in the workout routine.

Breathing:

No notes. Make sure to breathe softly if possible and avoid holding your breath as you do the movement as it would tense your body.

Note:

As you perform the movement, make sure to keep your hips up and not lower them down. By the end of the exercise, you will feel your glutes quite sore...that's normal, and very beneficial for sculpting your body!

WALL TRICEP PUSH-UP + KNEE RAISE

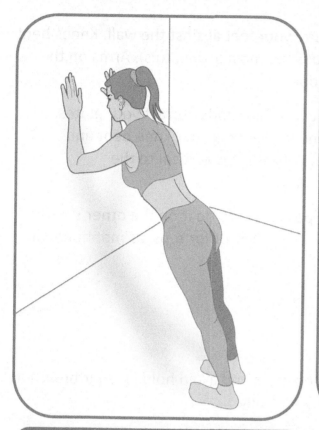

Step 1 - Perform Tricep Push-up

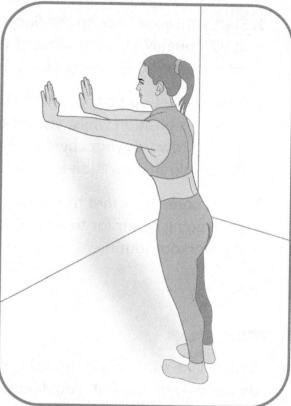

Step 2 - Come back into starting position.

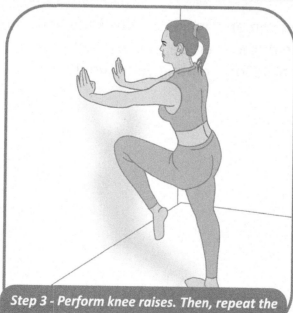

Step 3 - Perform knee raises. Then, repeat the whole sequence lifting the other leg.

How to do it:

1. Stand in front of a wall and place your hands on it shoulder-width apart. Stand roughly at an arm distance from it.

2. Then, perform a triceps push-up (pag. 21), bringing your forearm in touch with the wall.

3. Once you performed the triceps push-up and came back into the starting position, lift one thigh parallel to the floor. Hold 1'' and come back into the initial position.

4. Then, repeat the sequence, lifting the other thigh. Keep going with as many reps as mentioned in the workout plan.

Breathing:

The advice is to inhale every time you come back into the initial position, and exhale once you do the effort, so when you lift the thigh and perform the triceps push-up. Bear in mind that you do not have to necessarily think about how to breath here. I would suggest applying this tip in case you feel your breathing pattern is wrong.

Breathe naturally if you feel comfortable doing so.

Note:

Great combo to work different areas of your body to tone and sculpt many muscles at the same time. To make it more challenging, perform the sequence faster.

WALL STANDING MOUNTAIN CLIMBER

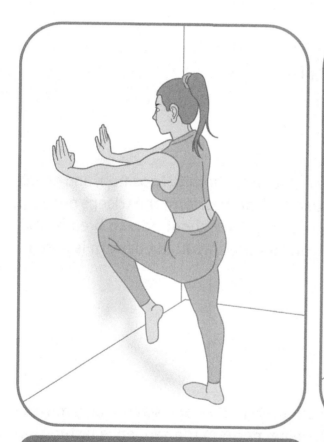

Step 1 – Lift one knee with thighs (at least) parallel to the floor.

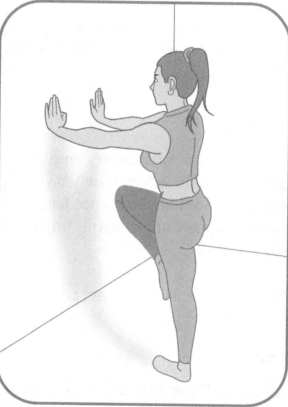

Step 2 – Come back into starting position and repeat with the other leg.

How to do it:

1. Stand facing a wall with feet hip width apart and hands shoulder width on the wall.

2. Whilst keeping your trunk straight, lift one leg with your knee at least parallel to the floor.

3. Then, come back into starting position and repeat with the other leg (do it fast if you feel comfortable, otherwise start at your own comfortable rhythm).

Breathing:

No tips needed. Especially if you do it fast there will be no time to focus on the breathing pattern. However, inhaling through your nose and exhaling through your mouth or nose is always recommended.

Note:

Feel free to do it at high-speed bouncing on the spot and only staying on the ball of your feet if you feel comfortable and your fitness level allows it. Otherwise, if you are not familiar with this exercise simply start taking a step each time, coming back into the initial position, and repeat. I can assure you that in a few sessions you will feel much lighter and more energized.

EXTEND GLUTE
BRIDGE + ROTATION

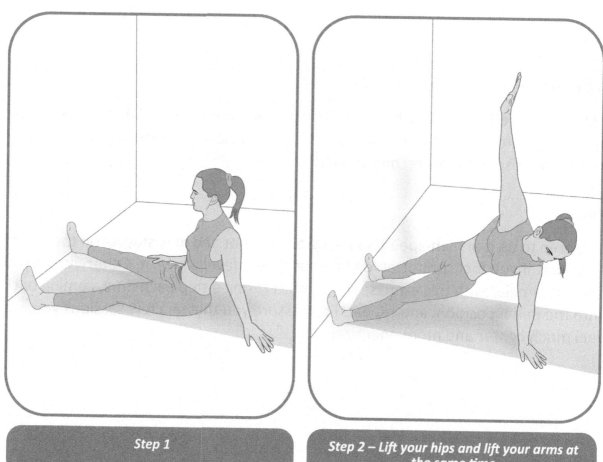

Step 1

Step 2 – Lift your hips and lift your arms at the same time

How to do it:

1. Sit in front of a wall with legs straight spread apart and feet against the wall. Place your left hand behind your body slightly to the side. Keep your trunk straight and chest up.

2. From this position, whilst keeping both arms and legs straight, lift your glutes off the floor as high as you can and extend your right arm over the ceiling.

3. Hold that position for 1'', and then return into the starting position. Once you perform all designed reps on one side, repeat it on the other side.

Breathing:

Exhale as you lift your hips. Inhale as you come back into the starting position with legs on the floor.

Note:

Make sure to breathe out as you extend your hips. Always keep your legs straight, applying pressure with your heels on the floor. Also, keep them against the wall to avoid slipping away from it.

Hey, don't forget you can **book your free 1-on-1 Wall Pilates session with me!** Just shoot an email with '**FREE CALL**' to avfitness99coaching@gmail.com and let's set up a training session together!

FULL BODY FOCUS

EXTENDED
DOWNWARD PLANK

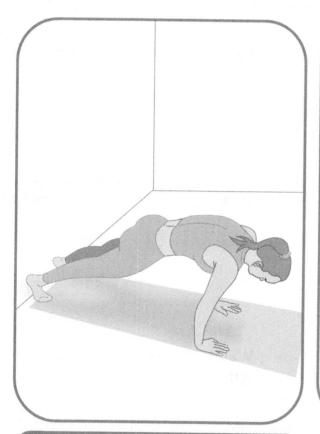

Step 1 – Plank with arms straight

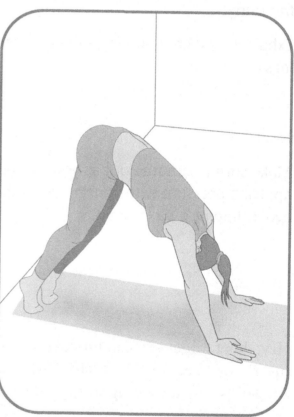

Step 2 - Lift your glutes up in a V-shape

How to do it:

1. Start by place yourself in a plank position, keeping your arms straight. Soles of your feet against with the wall. Keep your body straight.

2. From this position raise your hips to form a V-shape with your body (the so-called Downward Dog position). Keep your legs and arms straight as you do so (minimal bend at the knee is allowed).

3. Hold it for a second, and then come back into the plank position. Repeat for the mentioned reps.

Breathing:

Exhale as you lift your hips from plank to downward dog position. Inhale as you come back into the plank position (the starting position).

Note:

Make sure to keep your body in a straight line from your ankles up to your shoulders. You should not feel anything on your low back. All the tension should be on your core and a bit on your shoulders and front of your thighs.

When you lift your hips, you will feel a nice stretch on your back and shoulders. Keep your arms straight as you do so to make the exercise more effective.

When you lower down into the starting position (plank with arms straight) do not go too low with your hips. This is a common mistake that might cause low back pain.

WALL TRICEP PUSH-UP

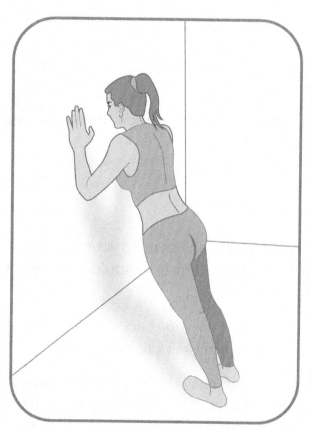

Starting position – Forearms on the wall.

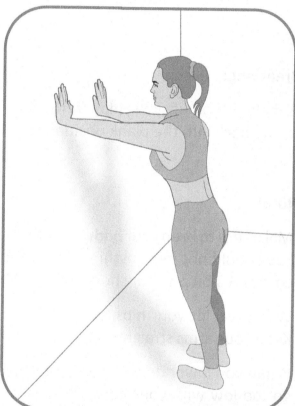

Final position – Hands only on the wall. Then repeat for mentioned reps.

How to do it:

1. Stand facing the wall two to three feet away from it. Place your forearm shoulder-width apart against it as shown in the image.

2. By pressing with your hands on the wall, lift your elbows so that your arms are going to be in a straight position.

3. Then, slowly come back into the starting position with forearms on the wall, and repeat for the mentioned reps.

Breathing:

No major tips needed. Ideally, you would inhale as you lower down into starting position and exhale as you push with your hands against the wall.

Note:

Great exercise to tone your arms and avoid the "bingo wings". Many of my female clients love this exercise as it really feels like the skin on the back of the arm is getting tighter just after one session!

To make the exercise slightly easier, come closer to the wall with your body and/or bring your hands in line with your head, so slightly higher than shown in the image.

Instead, to make it more challenging, step back and /or bring your hands slightly lower than your shoulders.

WALL PUSH-UP

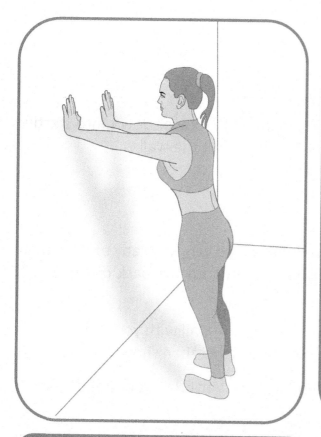

Step 1 – Starting position.

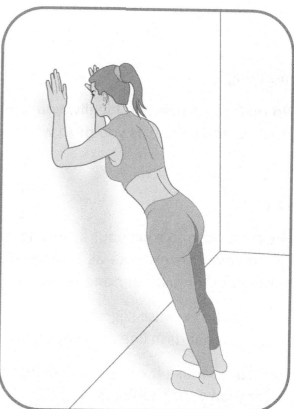

Step 2 – Lean forward and bend your elbows. Then, push back up into the starting position.

How to do it:

1. Stand facing the wall at arm distance from it.

2. Place your hands on the wall slightly wider than shoulder width. Feet slightly apart. In this position you will be slightly leaning towards the wall.

3. Whilst keeping your body in a straight line, bend your arms and lean forward with your chest almost touching the wall. Make sure to keep your elbows quite close to your trunk instead of lifting them out wide.

4. Then, push back up into the starting position by pushing the wall with your hands. You will feel the arms muscle doing most of the effort.

5. Repeat for the mentioned reps.

Breathing:

Ideally, you would inhale as you are leaning towards the wall, and then quickly exhale (through your mouth) as you push back up into the starting position.

Note:

It is quite common to bend at the hips as you lean forward and /or flare out the elbows on the side. Avoid these two mistakes as they could make the exercise less effective. Push-ups are a great exercise to tone your arms and shoulders as well as toning your core...Take advantage of it!

Also, once you lean forward, you might find yourself on the ball of your feet. That's ok.

KNEELING CHEST RAISE

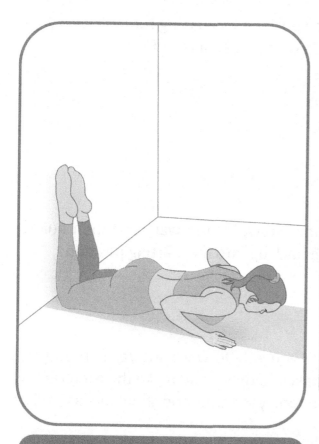

Step 1 – Starting position

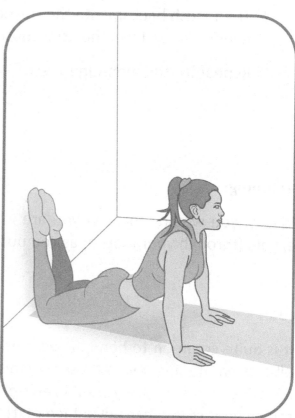

Step 2 – Half push-up and open your chest.

How to do it:

1. Place yourself close to the wall with your belly in touch with the floor (or a mat, preferably). Place your hands next to your shoulders quite close to your body. Knees will be in contact with the floor and shins against the wall.

2. From this position lift your chest and head assisting yourself with your arms. Exhale fully through the nose or mouth for 2'' as you perform the movement.

3. Then, return into the starting position, and repeat. As you return into the starting position inhale softly through your nose.

Breathing:

In this exercise, the breathing pattern is important. The inhaling and exhaling phases have already been mentioned. Also, avoid holding your breath as, for some people, it comes naturally doing so, especially when doing a new exercise that their body is not used to doing.

Note:

Make sure to perform this exercise slowly and in a controlled way. This is great to mobilize your spine, improve your posture and tone your upper body.

Once you lift your chest, try to bring your shoulders down, avoiding shrugging (Basically, think to create space between shoulders and ears).

WALL HIP THRUST

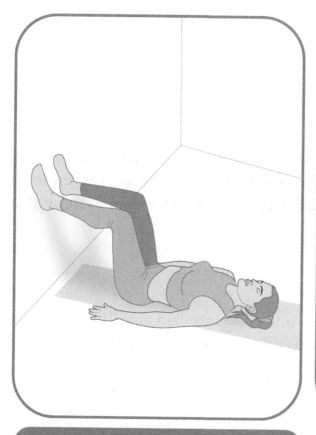

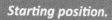
Starting position.

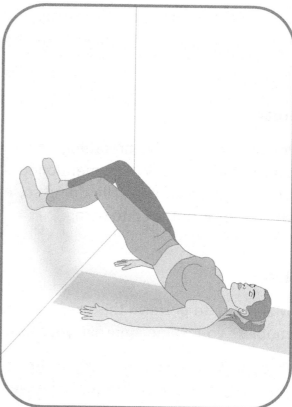
Final position- Squeeze your glutes as you do so.

How to do it:

1. Start with your back on the floor and your feet on the wall. Knees bent at 90°. Arms on the side of your body.

2. From this position bring your hips up and squeeze your glutes as you lift your hips.

3. Then, come back into starting position and repeat for the mentioned reps in the workout routine.

Breathing:

Exhale via your mouth as you lift your hips. Inhale as you come back into the initial position.

Note:

Ideally you want to be at 90° at the knees and at the hip joint.

When performing the exercise, bring your glutes up and squeeze them as you do so. This way you are not only engaging them but also preventing injuries and pain in your low back. Stronger and more toned glutes mean that your low back is protected too! If at any moment you feel your low back painful, it means probably the technique is not correct.

Focus on closing your hips (do the opposite of arching your low back) and contract both glutes and core as you do so. Some of my clients have had that same problem and by applying this cue the low back ache disappeared!

WALL KICK BACK

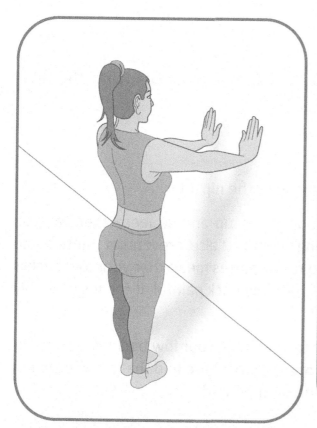

Starting position.

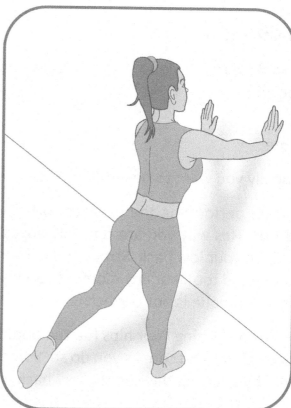

Final position – Hold it for 1" and come back
into the starting position.

How to do it:

1. Stand facing the wall two feet apart from it. Extend your arms in front of you and place them against the wall shoulder-width apart.

2. Lift your left leg and kick it straight behind your body. Hold this position for 1''.

3. Then, come back into the starting position and repeat for the mentioned reps. Then, perform it on the other side.

Breathing:

Exhale via your nose or mouth as you lift your leg. Inhale softly as you come back into the starting position.

Note:

Great exercise to improve your balance and tone the back of your leg. Some people prefer to stand a bit further from the wall so that their trunk is leaned forward. If that's you too, do it this way.

WALL GLUTE BRIDGE
HALF-ASSISTED

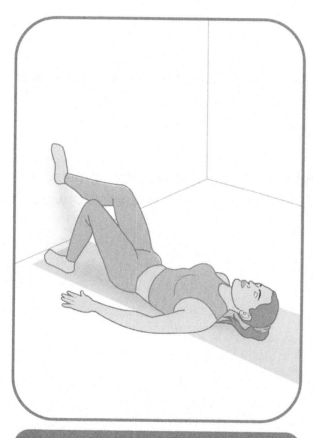

Starting position.

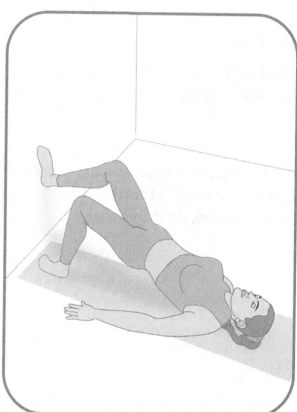

Final position – Hold the contraction for 1"

How to do it:

1. Lay down next to a wall with your right foot on it (and knee bent at 90° roughly) whilst the left one is planted on the floor with toes against the wall. Hands on the side.

2. From here, apply most of the pressure on the right foot to lift your hips. Hold the contraction on top for 2'' (Use the left foot on the floor just as assistance).

3. Lastly, come back slowly into the starting position and repeat for the mentioned reps. Then, switch sides.

Breathing:

As you squeeze your glutes and lift your hips exhale. Instead, inhale as you are resetting into the starting position.

Note:

Great variation that allows you to work on side at the time but still giving some work to the other leg. When I do a 1-on-1 session, people love this variation as they really feel like their legs and waistline are working and getting toned!

WALL CALF RAISES

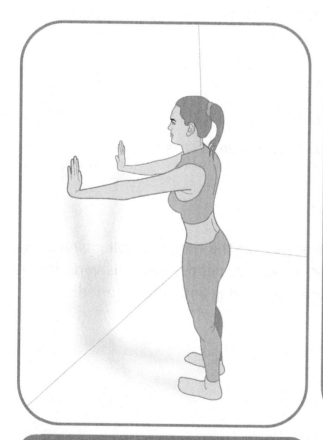

Starting position.

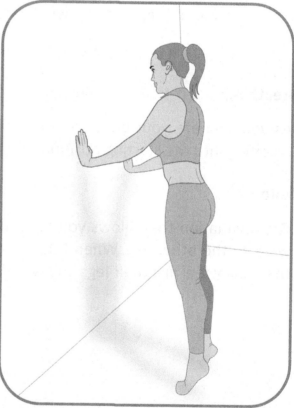

Final position – Hold the contraction for 1".

How to do it:

1. Stand in front of a wall and place your hands on it for assistance.

2. From here, lift your heels as high as you can by applying pressure with the ball of your feet to the ground.

3. Hold the contraction for 1'', and then come back into the starting position. Repeat the mentioned reps in the workout plan.

Breathing:

Exhale as you lift your toes, and then inhale as you lower down.

Note:

Keep your knees straight so that all the tension goes to the lower leg. It is a great exercise not only to tone the lower leg muscles, but also to strengthen the ankle and your feet, the first point of contact in any activities we do in our life!

WALL LATERAL LUNGE

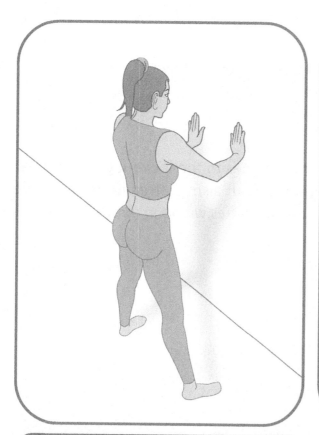

Starting position.

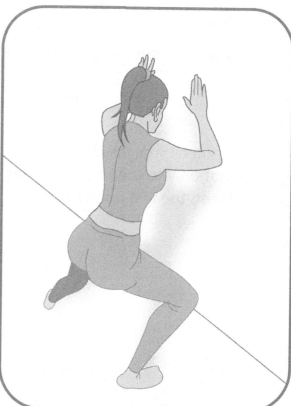

Final position — Lunge on one side, then repeat, come back into the starting position, and repeat on the other side.

How to do it:

1. Stand in front of the wall with hands against it at shoulder height. Spread your legs as you feel comfortable (as shown in the image would be perfect).

2. Whilst keeping the left leg straight and right foot pointing at the wall, bend your right knee and lower down in that direction, whilst keeping your trunk straight.

3. Once you get your hips roughly in line with your right knee (even with hips a bit higher as shown in the image works well) stop for a moment, and then come back into starting position. Then, repeat on the other side.

Breathing:

Inhale as you lower down on one side, and exhale as you come back into the starting position.

Note:

Ideally you would keep both feet pointing at the wall. This way you are going to stretch the inner thighs as well as working on ankle mobility, making this exercise very complete. However, if that's not possible and you feel uncomfortable doing so, feel free to lift your toes and point it outwards.

WALL LEG LIFTS

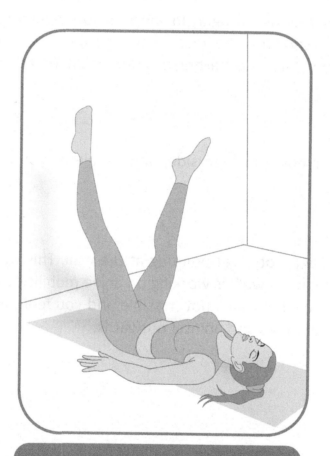

Lift one leg. Then, repeat on the other side.

How to do it:

1. Lay with your back on the floor as close as possible to the wall, with legs straight against it. Arms on the side.

2. Point your toes towards the ceiling and move one leg away from the wall. Hold it for 1''.

3. Then, come back into the starting position and repeat with the other leg.

Breathing:

No major tips are needed, breathe normally. The breath in this exercise does not impact the execution. Make sure not to hold your breath whilst moving.

Note:

Low-impact workout that can bring you benefits, especially if done towards the ends of the workout as it also helps to release some low back tension.

Hey, don't forget you can **book your free 1-on-1 Wall Pilates session with me!** Just shoot an email with **'FREE CALL'** to avfitness99coaching@gmail.com and let's set up a training session together!

WALL SQUATS

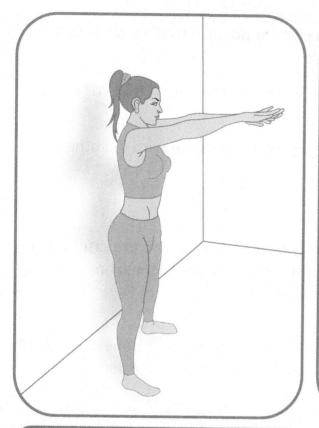

Step 1 – Stand next to a wall.

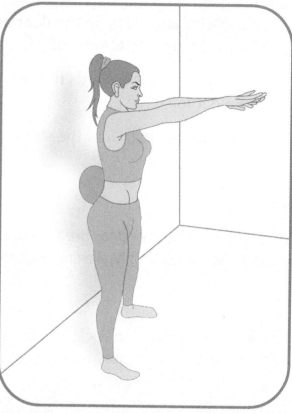

Step 1 (WITH THE BALL) - Stand next to a wall.

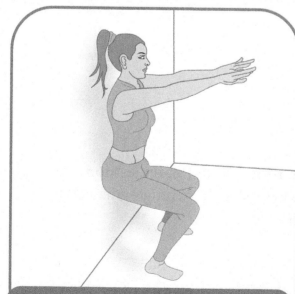

Step 2 (WITH THE BALL) -Squat down,
then push back up.

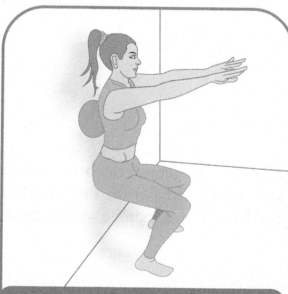

Step 2 (WITH THE BALL) -Squat down,
then push back up.

How to do it:

1. Stand with your back against the wall. Feel free to use a ball (small size or sponge ball works well) between your low back and the wall. As shown in the image, keep your arms straight in front of you.

2. Lower down slowly so that your thigh is roughly parallel to the floor. Then, hold for 1'' (The lower you go with squatting down, the harder it gets).

3. (As you lower down the ball will roll up towards the upper back)

4. Lastly, push back up into the starting position keeping your back in contact with the ball.

Breathing:

Inhale as you lower down, then breathe out as you stand back up again.

Note:

Feel free to use a small ball on your back so that you can roll down. Even doing it with no ball and just standing very close to the wall works well. Look at the images to see both variations.

ISO LEG HOLD UNILATERAL

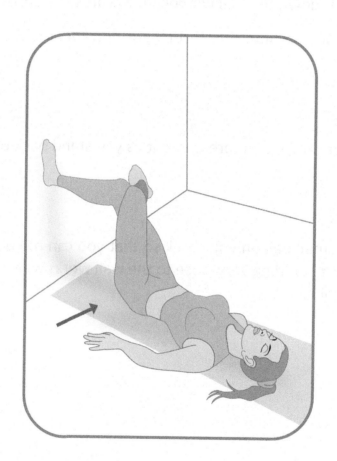

How to do it:

1. Lay down with your back on the floor and feet on the wall with your knees slightly bent. Arms on the side.

2. Place your left leg over your right thigh bending your knees, as shown in the image. Extend your hips.

3. Keep this position for the mentioned seconds whilst squeezing your glutes. Then, switch sides.

Breathing:

No tip is needed. Simply avoid holding your breath.

Note:

Push with your foot on the wall to activate the back of your leg. Focus on applying pressure with your heels on the wall to feel it more on your glutes.

This is a great exercise to tone up the back of your thighs and your butt without getting bulky.

WALL SPLIT SQUAT

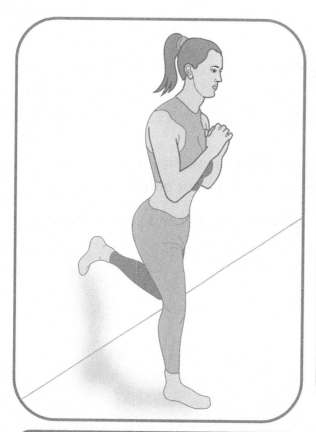

Starting position.

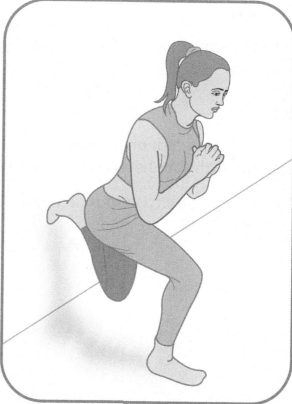

Final position – then push back up and repeat for reps. Then, switch sides.

How to do it:

1. Start balancing on your right leg having your left foot on the wall behind you at roughly thigh height. The initial position is very individual and so my suggestion is to play around until you find a comfortable setup (look at the image to have a clear idea on how it should look).

2. Keep your hands together in front of your chest.

3. Lower down putting most of your body weight on the front leg until your thigh is parallel to the floor (ideally, even a few inches above parallel works well). The right foot is pressed against the wall to help you with maintaining balance.

4. Hold the bottom position for 1-2'' and repeat for the desired reps. Then, switch sides.

Breathing:

Inhale softly as you lower down, and exhale quickly as you push back up into starting position.

Note:

Lower body burns guaranteed!

If you have experience with regular split squats, the setup is the same but the back foot instead of resting on a bench is pressing hard on the wall behind you.

Forward lean of your trunk is normal. The more you lean forward the more you are going to engage your glutes. The more you stay upright the more you will engage the front of your thighs.

SINGLE LEG WALL GLUTE BRIDGE

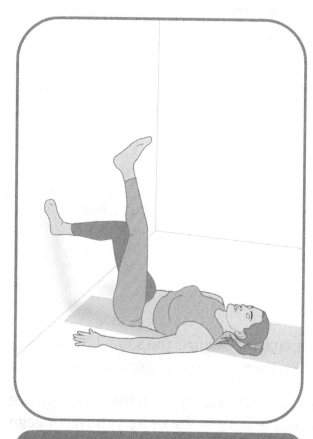

Starting Position

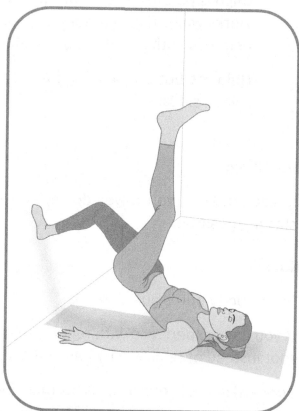

Final Position – Hold that position for 1", then come back into the starting position and repeat.

How to do it:

1. Start with back on the floor one to two feet distant from the wall and feet on the wall (Knees bent roughly at 90°).

2. From there lift your left leg in the air so that it is vertical to the ground.

3. Then, lift your hips by pushing with your right foot on the wall. Hold the contraction on top for 1''.

4. Lastly, come back into the starting position and repeat for the mentioned reps. Repeat on the other side.

Breathing:

Exhale fully as you lift your hips. Then, inhale as you are lowering down into the starting position.

Note:

If you want to feel more your glutes apply more pressure with your heel on the wall as well as go closer to the wall with your body. Instead, if you want to target the back of your thighs more, keep your whole foot on the wall and get a bit further from the wall, with the knee angle more than 90°.

CORE FOCUS

WALL LATERAL CRUNCH

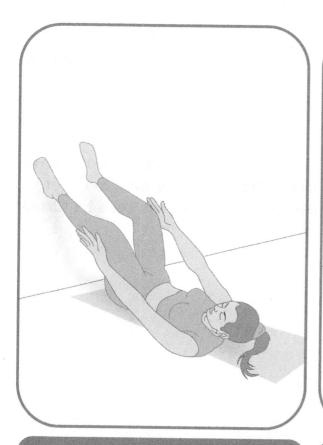

Step 1 - Starting position.

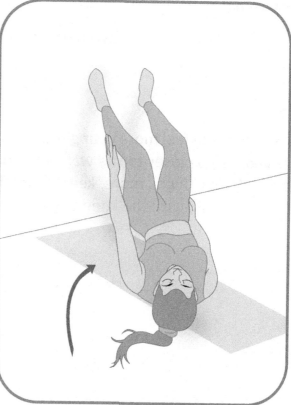

Step 2 – Bend on one side. Then, come back into the starting position and perform it on the other side.

How to do it:

1. Lay down with your low back on the floor (or on a mat, if more comfortable) and have your feet against the wall. Keep the knees bent at 90°. Arms on the side without touching the floor.

2. From there, slightly lift your upper back and then move your body on the left side so that your left hand almost touches the wall.

3. Then, come back into the starting position, and perform it on the other side.

Breathing:

As you bend towards the side, exhale quickly through your nose or mouth. Then when you come back into the starting position, inhale via your nose.

Note:

Great exercise to work on the obliques and tone the side area of your abs. Make sure to bend on the side to feel a contraction on the side abs. I always suggest to my 1-on-1 clients to keep their heads up and facing forward. However, for some clients this can be slightly uncomfortable. In that case, I would suggest to keep your head just slightly off the floor and look at the ceiling.

A common mistake is to perform this exercise fast. There is no need for it. Perform it at your own pace so that you can feel it well on the side of your abs.

WALL TWIST

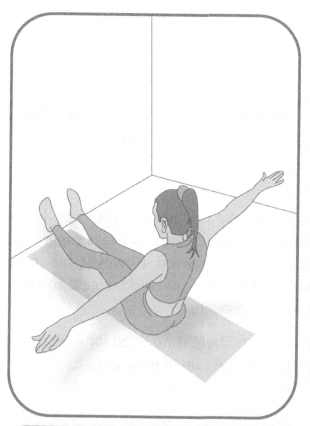

Step 1 – Starting position.

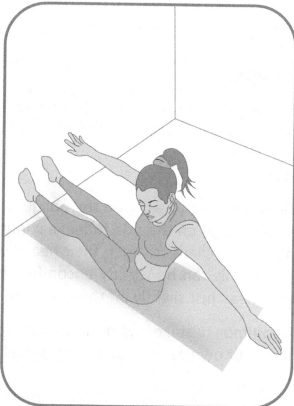

Step 2 – Rotate on one side, then come back into the starting position and do it on the other side.

How to do it:

1. Start by sitting in front of a wall with legs straight slightly lifted off the floor. Keep the sole of your feet on the wall. Also, spread out wide your arms and keep your body straight.

2. From this position, rotate towards one side. Hold the position for 1''.

3. Lastly, come back into the initial position and rotate to the other side. Repeat for the mentioned reps.

Breathing:

As you rotate towards right or left you exhale all the air through your mouth.

Once you are in the starting position take a soft inhale via your nose.

Note:

Great core exercise to tone your waist and make it slimmer. However, there is a small percentage of people that feel discomfort in their low back when performing this exercise. If you feel so, stop immediately and try it again in the future.

As an alternative you can try doing Wall Lateral Crunch (previous exercise).

SIT UPS STRAIGHT LEGGED

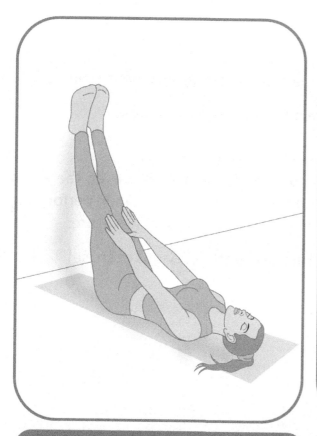

Step 1- Starting position.

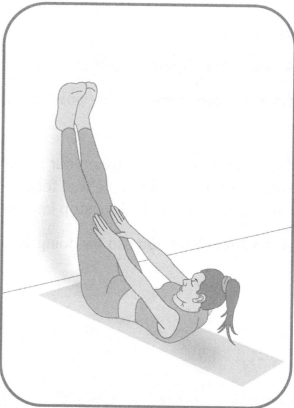

Step 2 - Final position. Then, repeat

How to do it:

1. Lie down on the floor (or mat, preferably) as close as possible to a wall. Lift your legs keeping them straight and place your heels on the wall. Hands on the side (See Step 1 for perfect starting position).

2. Try to touch your ankles with your hands whilst keeping your arms straight. By doing that you will do a crunch working all the muscle in your abs.

3. Then, come back into the starting position and repeat for the mentioned reps.

Breathing:

No tips needed.

Note:

To make it slightly easier you can distance the glutes from the wall a bit more and shorten the range of motion. It Is important to lift your upper back so that you crunch your abs. The lower back stays in contact with the floor the whole time.

For some people they experience the mat slipping away, making the exercise less effective. However, if you perform the exercise slowly, not only will you work your abs more (especially if you hold the contraction for 1"+) but also will limit this problem.

PLANK WALL TOUCHES

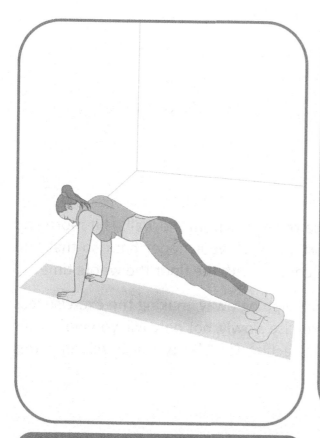

Step 1- Starting position.

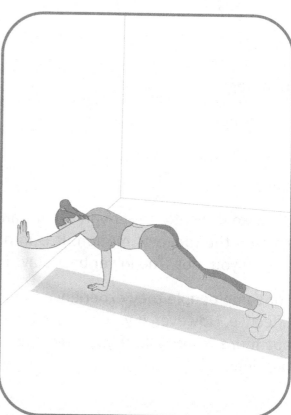

Step 2 – Touch with one hand the wall, then come back into the starting position. Then, repeat on the other side.

How to do it:

1. Place yourself in a plank position with feet together and arms straight just below your shoulders. Position your body at one arm distance from the wall.

2. Lift one hand from the floor and tap on the wall in front of you, whilst keeping your trunk straight.

3. Then, come back into the starting position, and repeat with the other hand. Keep alternating the two hands tapping the wall for the mentioned reps.

Breathing:

No big tips needed. Avoid just holding your breath as it would make the exercises less effective.

Note:

Avoid arching your back as you move your hands. Keep your back in a neutral position. Also, the tap is very quick. The slower you do it, the more difficult the exercise will become.

WALL REVERSE CRUNCH

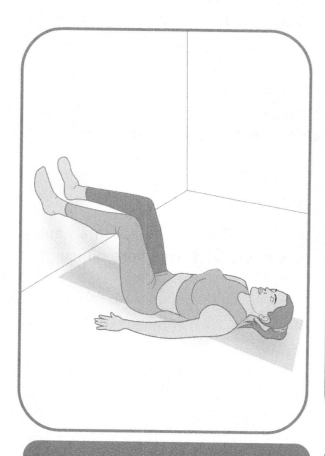

Step 1- Starting position.

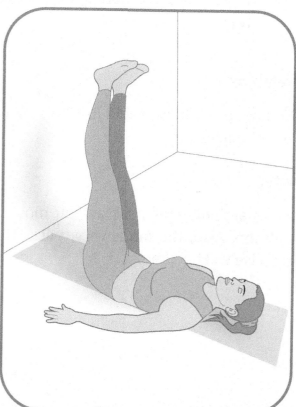

Step 2 – Lift legs towards you.
Then, repeat.

How to do it:

1. Lay down with your low back on a mat whilst having your feet against the wall. Keep the knees bent at 90°. Arms on the side in contact with the floor.

2. Bring your legs up and towards your chest whilst keeping your low back on the floor (from the floor only the hips area is going to be lifted).

3. Then, come back into the starting position and repeat for the mentioned reps.

Breathing:

No major tips needed. Avoid holding your breath as it can cause fatigue before your abs muscles are tired.

Note:

Great exercise to tone your lower abs. Make sure to keep your low back on the floor as much as possible to avoid low back discomfort and activate your lower abs. You will also feel some tension on your thighs.

WALL SIDE CRUNCH

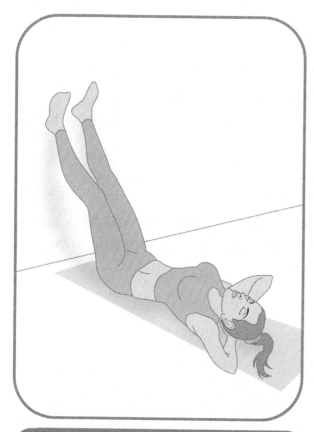

Starting position

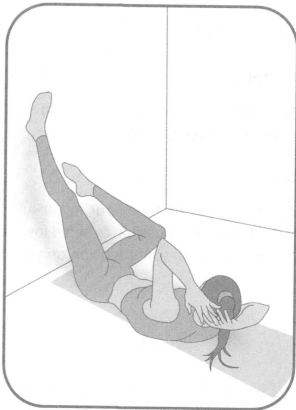

Final position – Lift upper back and reach knee with the opposite elbow. Repeat for reps, then switch sides.

How to do it:

1. Lay down close to a wall with your back on the floor. Position your feet on the wall with legs straight (bending your knees slightly works fine too) and hands behind your head.

2. From this position, perform a side crunch lifting your upper back. It means that you are going to bring your left elbow and right knee close together.

3. Lastly, come back into the starting position and repeat for the mentioned reps. Then, change sides.

Breathing:

Exhale as you perform the crunch. Inhale as you come back into the starting position.

Note:

Great exercise to tone your abs. Make sure that your low back is in contact with the floor so to avoid low back pain as well as activate your abs.

WALL WALKING PLANK

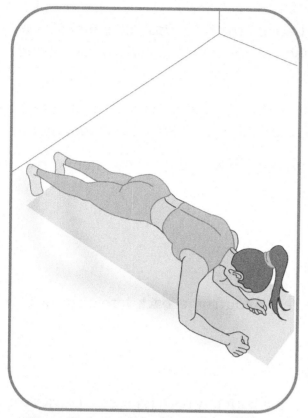

Step 1 – Starting position with legs on the floor

Step 2 – One leg straight up

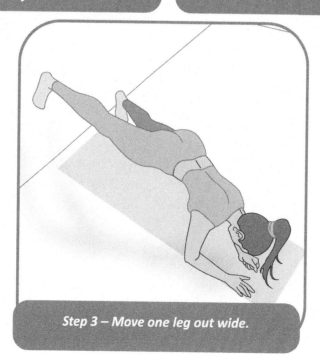

Step 3 – Move one leg out wide.

How to do it:

1. Get in a plank position with elbows just below your shoulders whilst keeping your body in a straight line. Position your feet very close to the wall (it doesn't have to touch it even though some people perform it with the sole of their feet against the wall).

2. Whilst keeping the plank position, lift your right leg straight up. Keep the position for just half a second.

3. Then, move it sideways without the need to touch the wall. Keep it for just half a second.

4. Lastly, come back into the starting position and repeat for the mentioned reps. Once you finish the reps with your right leg, perform them with the left leg moving.

Breathing:

No major tips needed. Avoid holding your breath as it can reduce your performance.

Note:

Amazing core exercise that you probably have done before. Make sure not to arch your low back but to keep your body in a straight line. The leg movement will increase the challenge.

If that's too easy do the movement slower and hold each step for a few seconds.

If that's too difficult just perform the movement and get through the steps quickly.

Over time, the goal is to master the whole sequence without any rush.

28-DAY CHALLENGE
THE ULTIMATE CHALLENGE FOR A TINY WAIST AND SCULPTING YOUR BODY.

This challenge will be a great start for your wall Pilates workouts! This has been proven on dozens of people I train 1-on-1, and everyone got some benefits with less than 20 minutes of exercise daily!

The main feedback I received from clients are:

• More Toned Abs

People felt their belly got flatter and more toned after just a few sessions (Obviously, their diet played a role too, I assume).

• Slimmer Waist

As you can see if you have already tried some of these exercises, you are going to sweat and burn calories. This will imply that you are going to get rid of some body fat, making your waist visibly slimmer in less than a month.

• Gained Strength and Balance

By doing full body routines you will notice more strength in all the exercises, translating to more strength in daily life activities.

• Improved Well-Being

As you probably know from your experience, exercises, such as Pilates, improves mental clarity and decreases anxiety and overthinking, as it will ground you in the present moment, moving your body in tune with your breathing patterns.

Note before starting: Try to do these exercises in sequence with minimal rest in between. When mentioned to perform "two to three sets", as an example, it means that after the last exercises you can rest anywhere between 30 to 60 seconds, and then repeat the whole sequence. I would not recommend you take longer breaks as it will lower the heart rate too much, making the workout less effective.

DAY 1 – Perform one to two sets

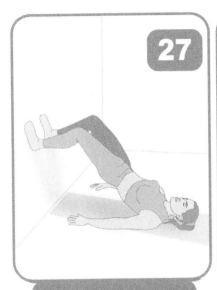

27

Wall Hip Thrust

10 repetitions

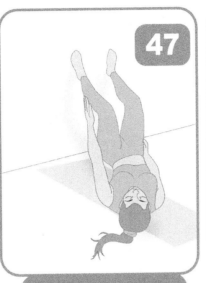

47

Wall Lateral Crunch

8 reps each side

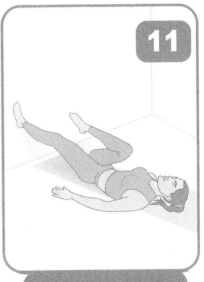

11

Wall Marches

6 reps each side(alternated) or 30'' work

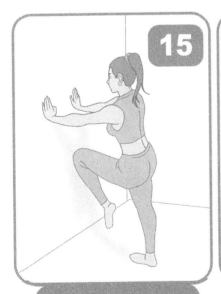

15

Wall Standing Moun tain Climber

30'' work

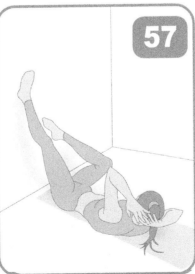

57

Wall Side Crunch

10 reps each side

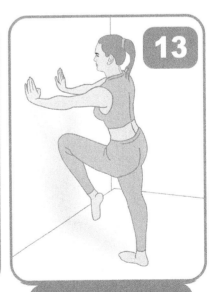

13

Wall Tricep Push-up + Knee Raise

10 reps (5 lifting left leg, 5 right one)

DAY 2 – Perform one to two sets

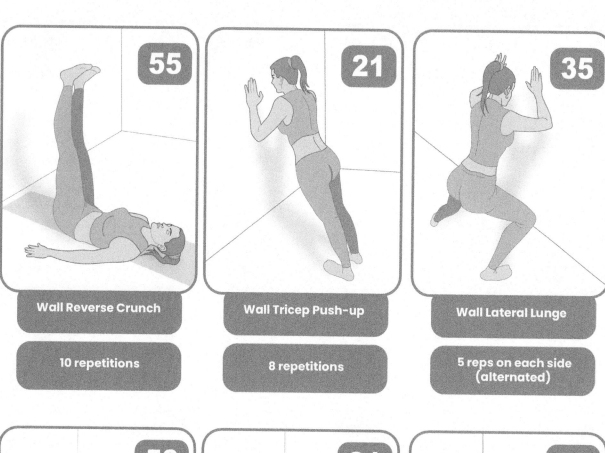

55 Wall Reverse Crunch
10 repetitions

21 Wall Tricep Push-up
8 repetitions

35 Wall Lateral Lunge
5 reps on each side (alternated)

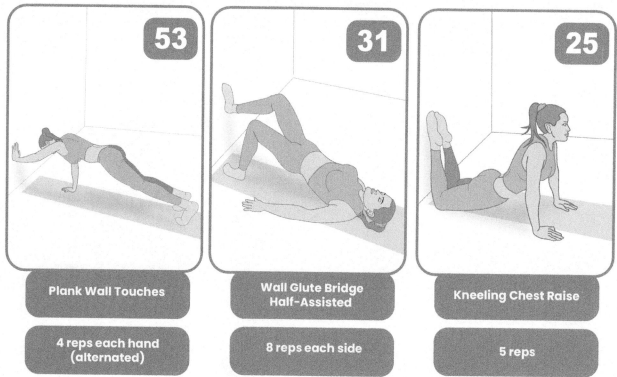

53 Plank Wall Touches
4 reps each hand (alternated)

31 Wall Glute Bridge Half-Assisted
8 reps each side

25 Kneeling Chest Raise
5 reps

DAY 3 – Perform one to two sets

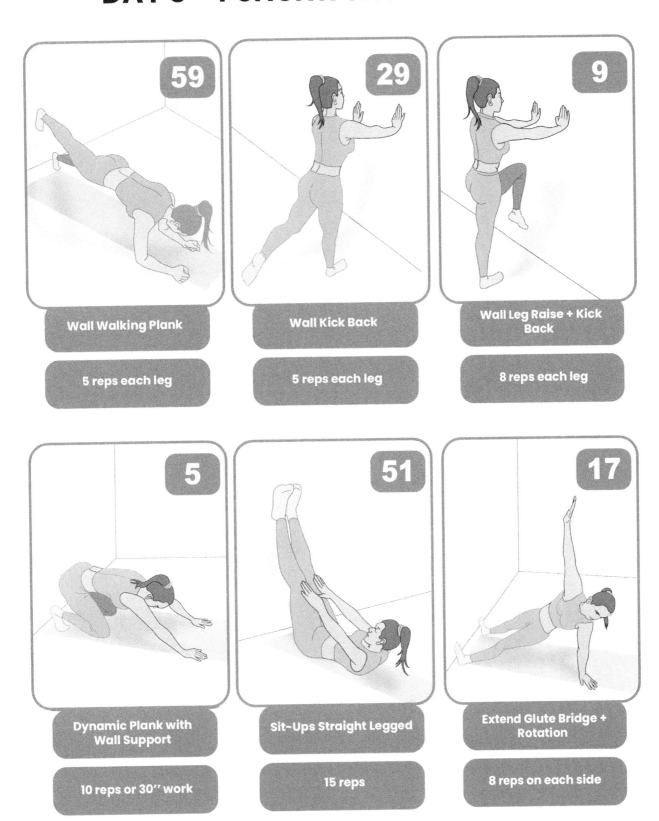

59

Wall Walking Plank

5 reps each leg

29

Wall Kick Back

5 reps each leg

9

Wall Leg Raise + Kick Back

8 reps each leg

5

Dynamic Plank with Wall Support

10 reps or 30'' work

51

Sit-Ups Straight Legged

15 reps

17

Extend Glute Bridge + Rotation

8 reps on each side

DAY 4 – Perform one to two sets

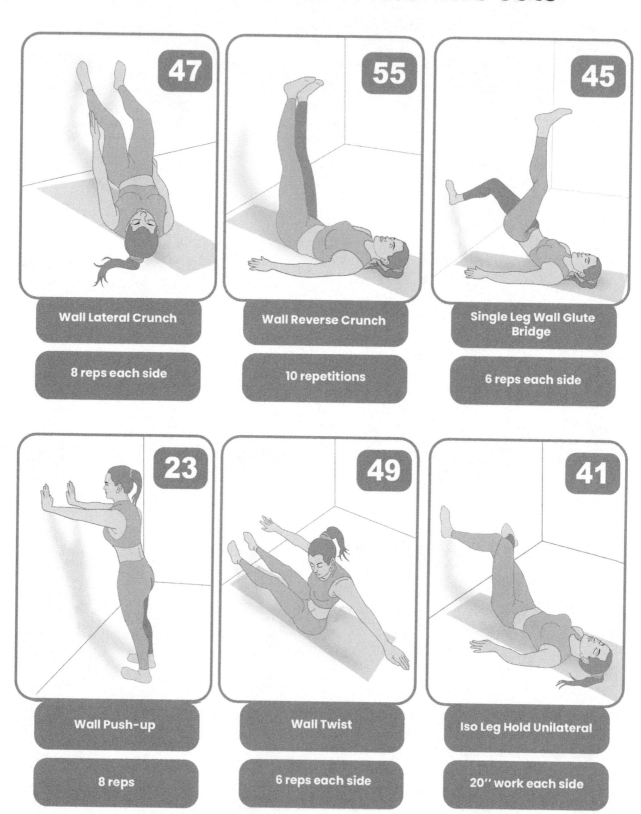

47 Wall Lateral Crunch — 8 reps each side

55 Wall Reverse Crunch — 10 repetitions

45 Single Leg Wall Glute Bridge — 6 reps each side

23 Wall Push-up — 8 reps

49 Wall Twist — 6 reps each side

41 Iso Leg Hold Unilateral — 20'' work each side

DAY 5 – Perform one to two sets

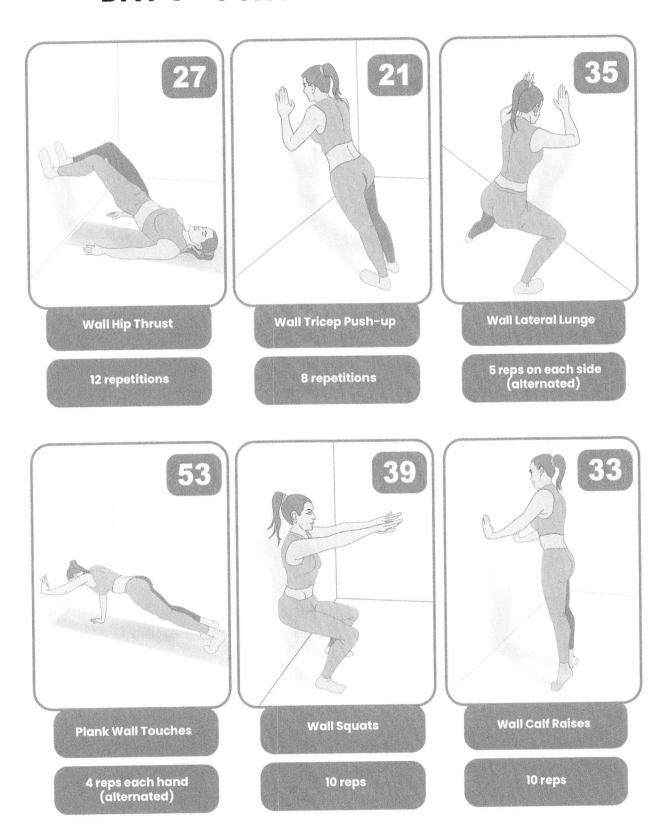

27

Wall Hip Thrust

12 repetitions

21

Wall Tricep Push-up

8 repetitions

35

Wall Lateral Lunge

5 reps on each side
(alternated)

53

Plank Wall Touches

4 reps each hand
(alternated)

39

Wall Squats

10 reps

33

Wall Calf Raises

10 reps

DAY 6 – Perform one to two sets

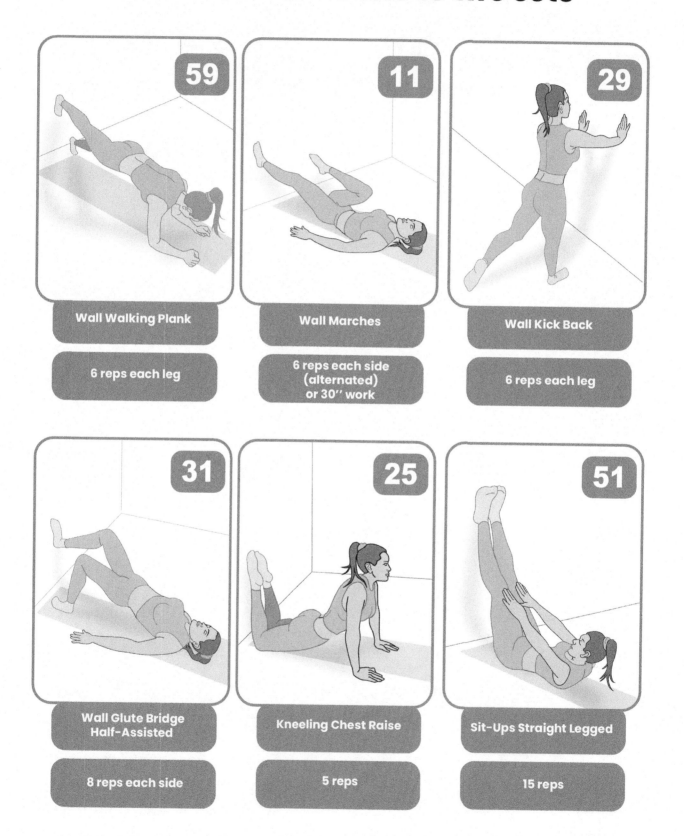

59
Wall Walking Plank

6 reps each leg

11
Wall Marches

6 reps each side
(alternated)
or 30'' work

29
Wall Kick Back

6 reps each leg

31
Wall Glute Bridge
Half-Assisted

8 reps each side

25
Kneeling Chest Raise

5 reps

51
Sit-Ups Straight Legged

15 reps

DAY 7 – Perform one to two sets

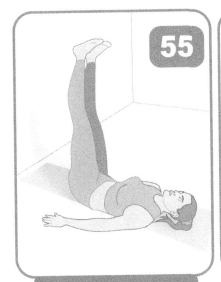

55

Wall Reverse Crunch

12 repetitions

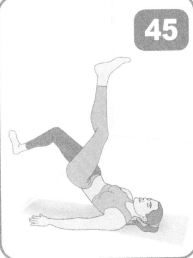

45

Single Leg Wall Glute Bridge

6 reps each side

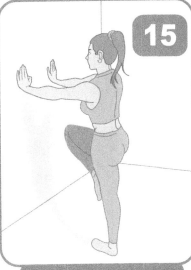

15

Wall Standing Mountain Climber

35" work

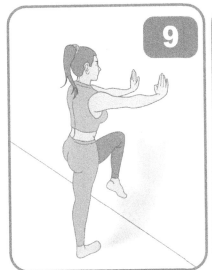

9

Wall Leg Raise + Kick Back

8 reps each leg

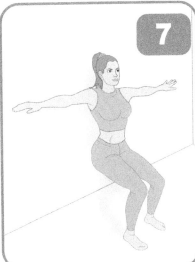

7

Wall Sit + Arm Circles

30" work
(Or 15 circles clockwise +
15 circles anticlockwise)

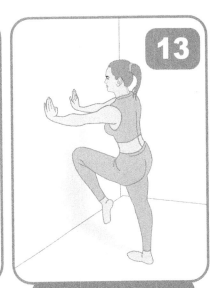

13

Wall Tricep push-up + Knee Raise

10 reps (5 lifting left leg, 5 right one)

DAY 8 – Perform one to two sets

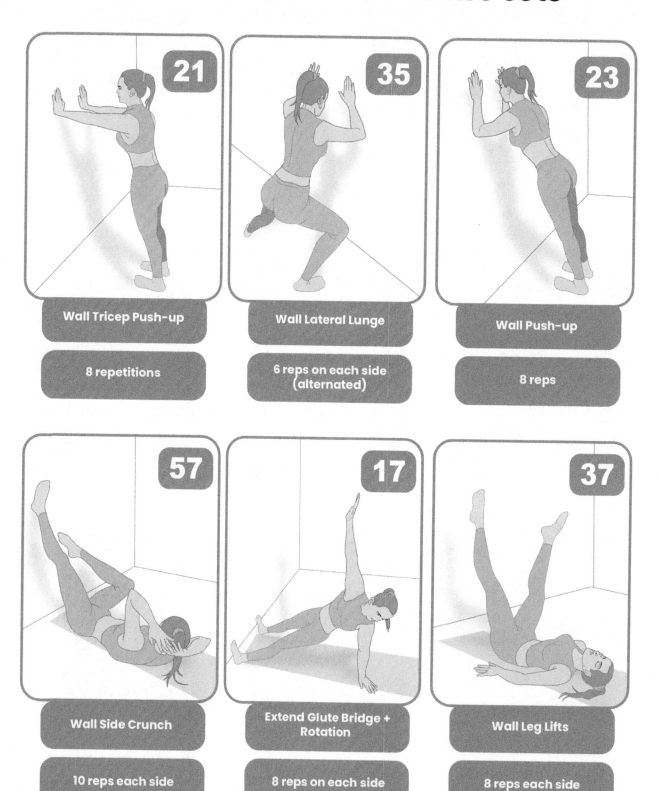

21
Wall Tricep Push-up
8 repetitions

35
Wall Lateral Lunge
6 reps on each side (alternated)

23
Wall Push-up
8 reps

57
Wall Side Crunch
10 reps each side

17
Extend Glute Bridge + Rotation
8 reps on each side

37
Wall Leg Lifts
8 reps each side

DAY 9 – Perform one to two sets

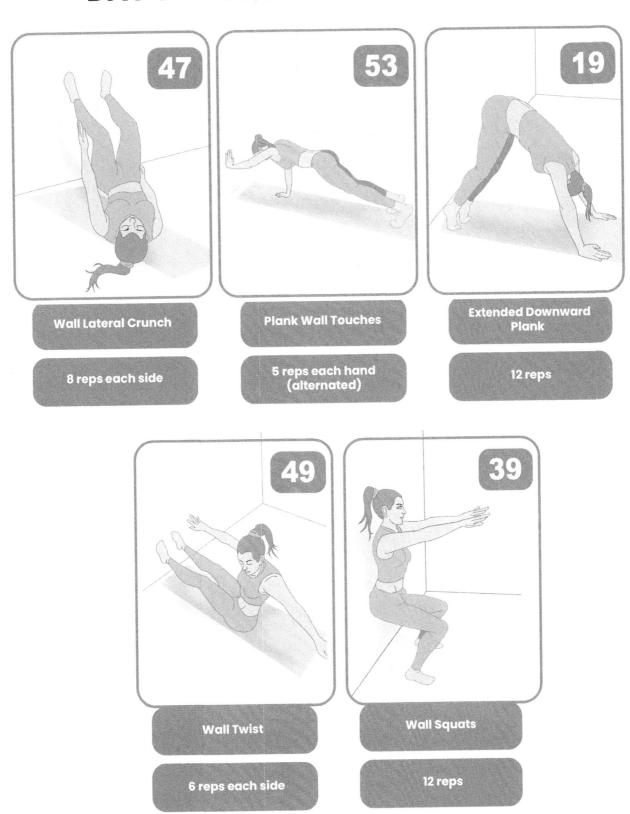

47

Wall Lateral Crunch

8 reps each side

53

Plank Wall Touches

5 reps each hand (alternated)

19

Extended Downward Plank

12 reps

49

Wall Twist

6 reps each side

39

Wall Squats

12 reps

DAY 10 – Perform one to two sets

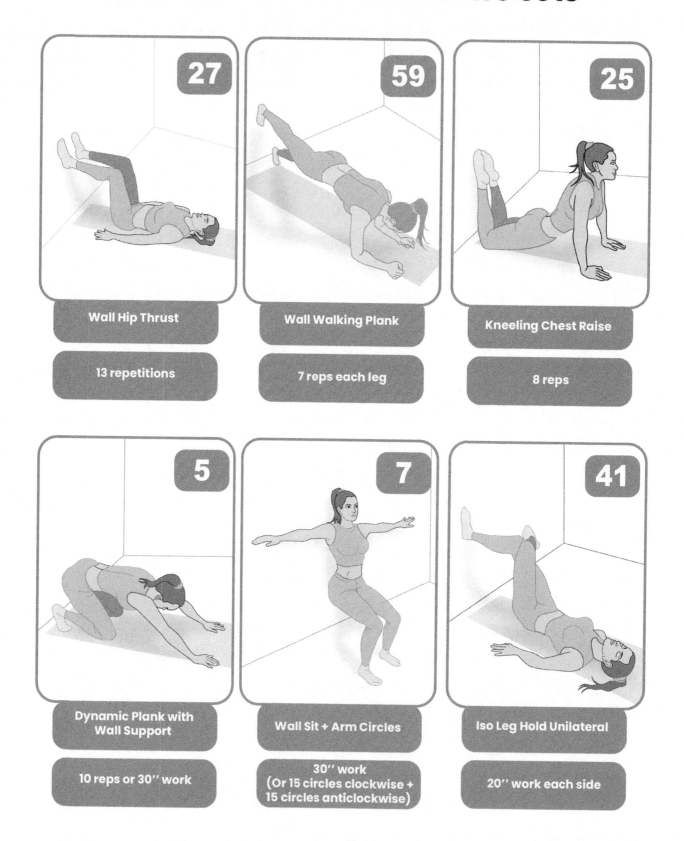

27

Wall Hip Thrust

13 repetitions

59

Wall Walking Plank

7 reps each leg

25

Kneeling Chest Raise

8 reps

5

Dynamic Plank with Wall Support

10 reps or 30'' work

7

Wall Sit + Arm Circles

30'' work
(Or 15 circles clockwise +
15 circles anticlockwise)

41

Iso Leg Hold Unilateral

20'' work each side

DAY 11 – Perform two to three sets

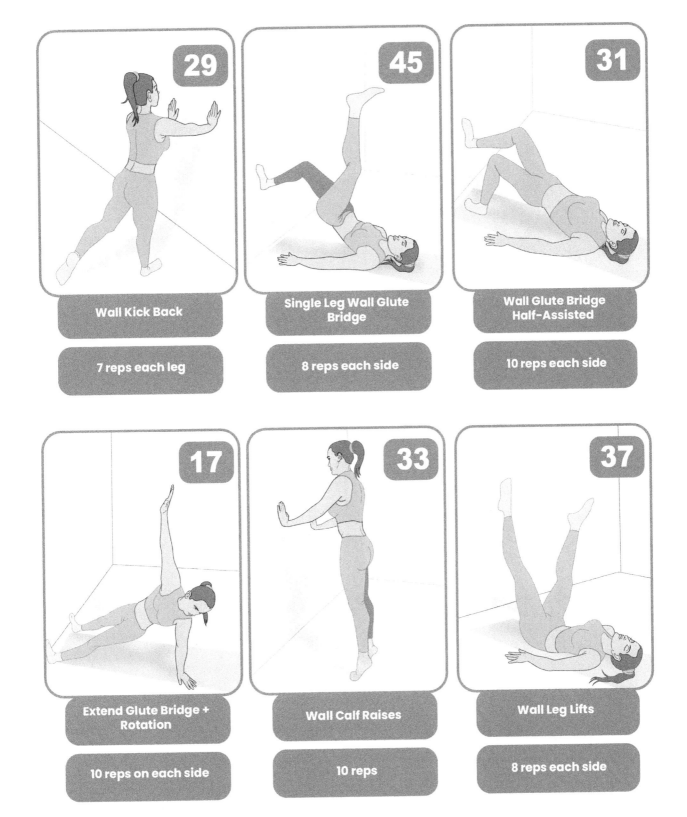

Wall Kick Back

7 reps each leg

Single Leg Wall Glute Bridge

8 reps each side

Wall Glute Bridge Half-Assisted

10 reps each side

Extend Glute Bridge + Rotation

10 reps on each side

Wall Calf Raises

10 reps

Wall Leg Lifts

8 reps each side

DAY 12 – Perform two to three sets

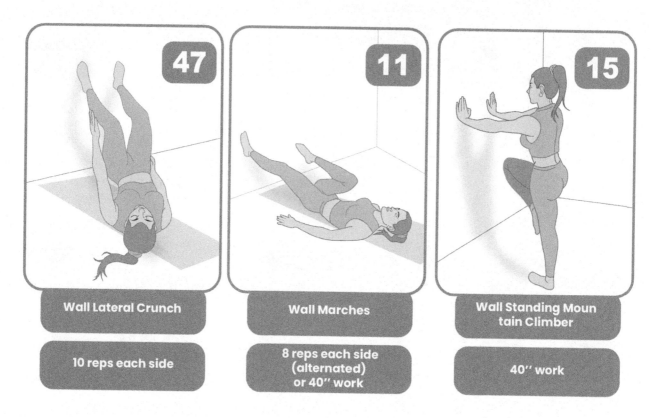

47

Wall Lateral Crunch

10 reps each side

11

Wall Marches

8 reps each side
(alternated)
or 40" work

15

**Wall Standing Moun
tain Climber**

40" work

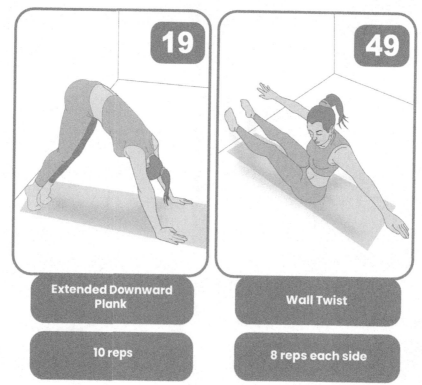

19

**Extended Downward
Plank**

10 reps

49

Wall Twist

8 reps each side

DAY 13 – Perform two to three sets

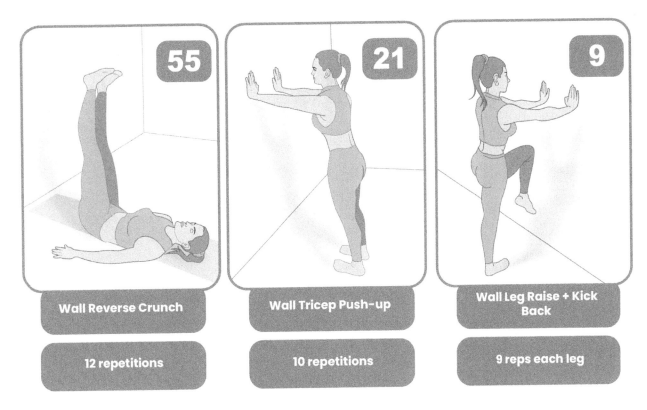

Wall Reverse Crunch

12 repetitions

Wall Tricep Push-up

10 repetitions

Wall Leg Raise + Kick Back

9 reps each leg

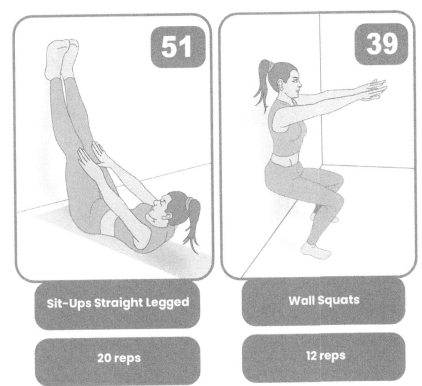

Sit-Ups Straight Legged

20 reps

Wall Squats

12 reps

DAY 14 – Perform two to three sets

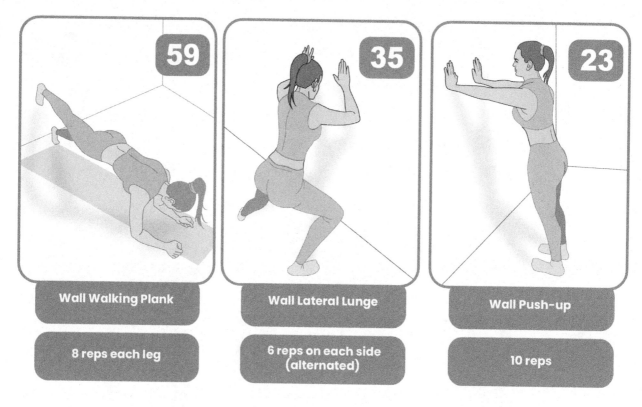

59

Wall Walking Plank

8 reps each leg

35

Wall Lateral Lunge

6 reps on each side
(alternated)

23

Wall Push-up

10 reps

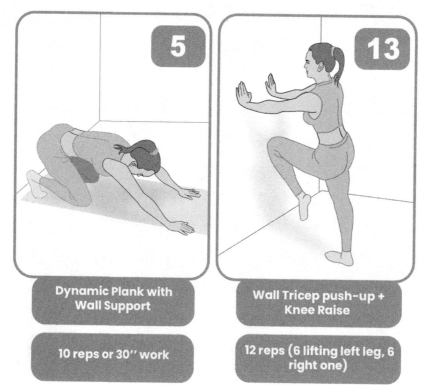

5

**Dynamic Plank with
Wall Support**

10 reps or 30″ work

13

**Wall Tricep push-up +
Knee Raise**

12 reps (6 lifting left leg, 6
right one)

DAY 15 – Perform two to three sets

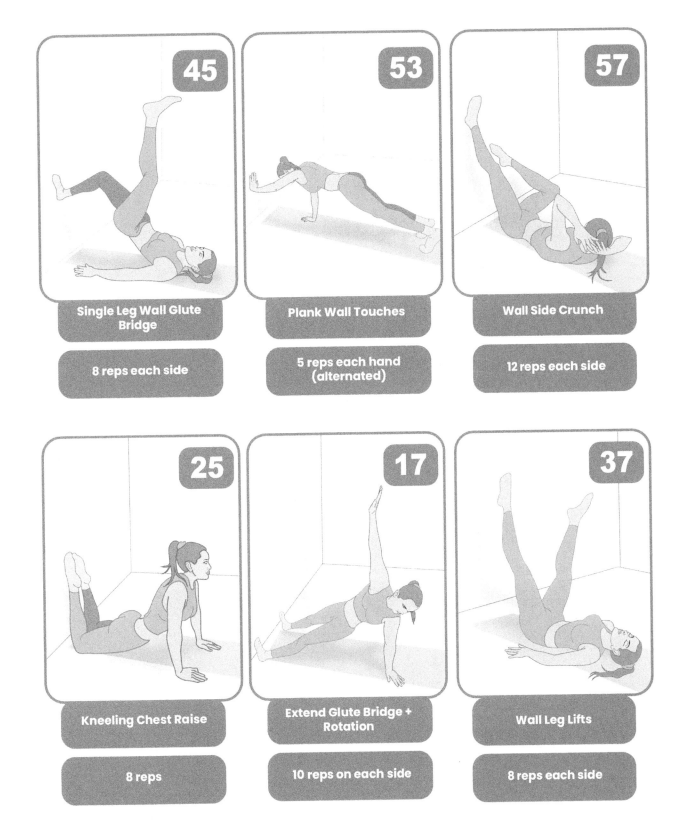

45

Single Leg Wall Glute Bridge

8 reps each side

53

Plank Wall Touches

5 reps each hand (alternated)

57

Wall Side Crunch

12 reps each side

25

Kneeling Chest Raise

8 reps

17

Extend Glute Bridge + Rotation

10 reps on each side

37

Wall Leg Lifts

8 reps each side

DAY 16 – Perform two to three sets

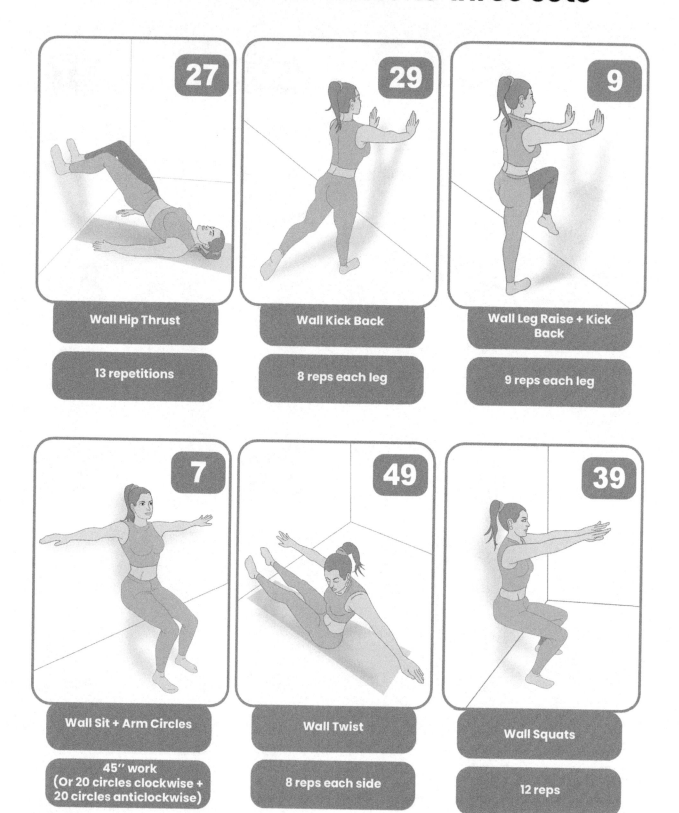

27
Wall Hip Thrust
13 repetitions

29
Wall Kick Back
8 reps each leg

9
Wall Leg Raise + Kick Back
9 reps each leg

7
Wall Sit + Arm Circles
45'' work
(Or 20 circles clockwise +
20 circles anticlockwise)

49
Wall Twist
8 reps each side

39
Wall Squats
12 reps

DAY 17 – Perform two to three sets

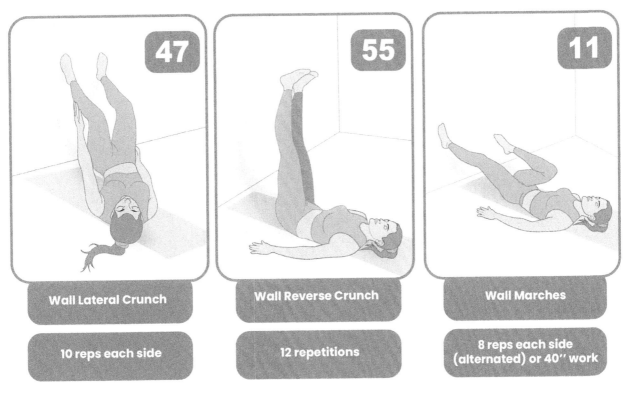

47

Wall Lateral Crunch

10 reps each side

55

Wall Reverse Crunch

12 repetitions

11

Wall Marches

8 reps each side (alternated) or 40'' work

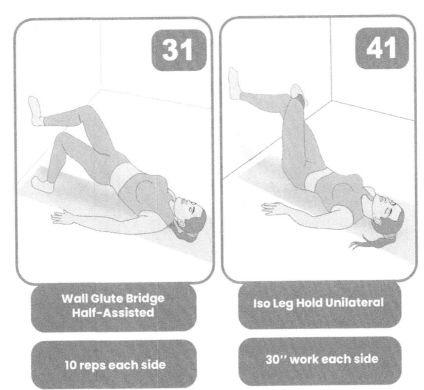

31

Wall Glute Bridge Half-Assisted

10 reps each side

41

Iso Leg Hold Unilateral

30'' work each side

DAY 18 – Perform two to three sets

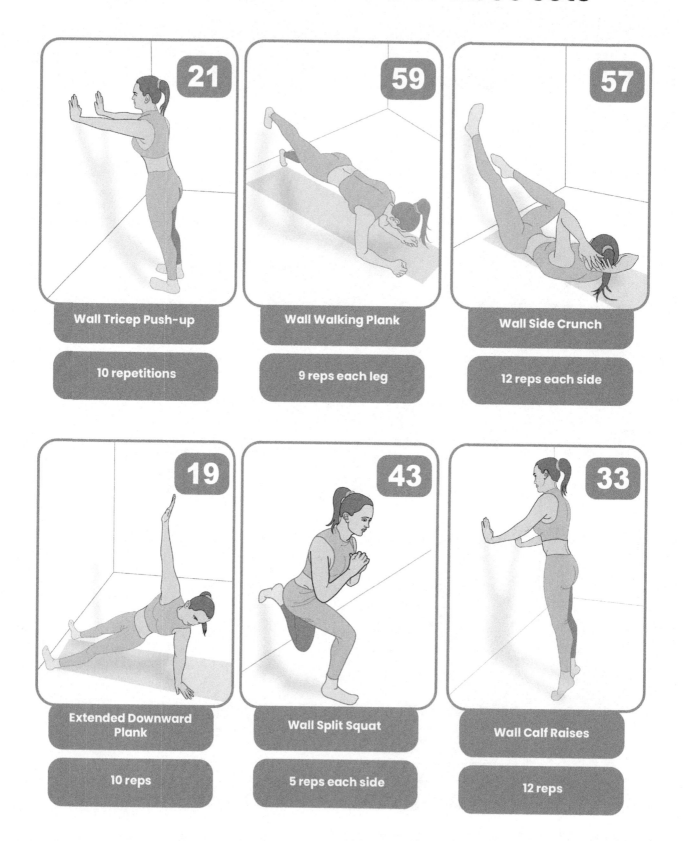

21

Wall Tricep Push-up

10 repetitions

59

Wall Walking Plank

9 reps each leg

57

Wall Side Crunch

12 reps each side

19

Extended Downward Plank

10 reps

43

Wall Split Squat

5 reps each side

33

Wall Calf Raises

12 reps

DAY 19 – Perform two to three sets

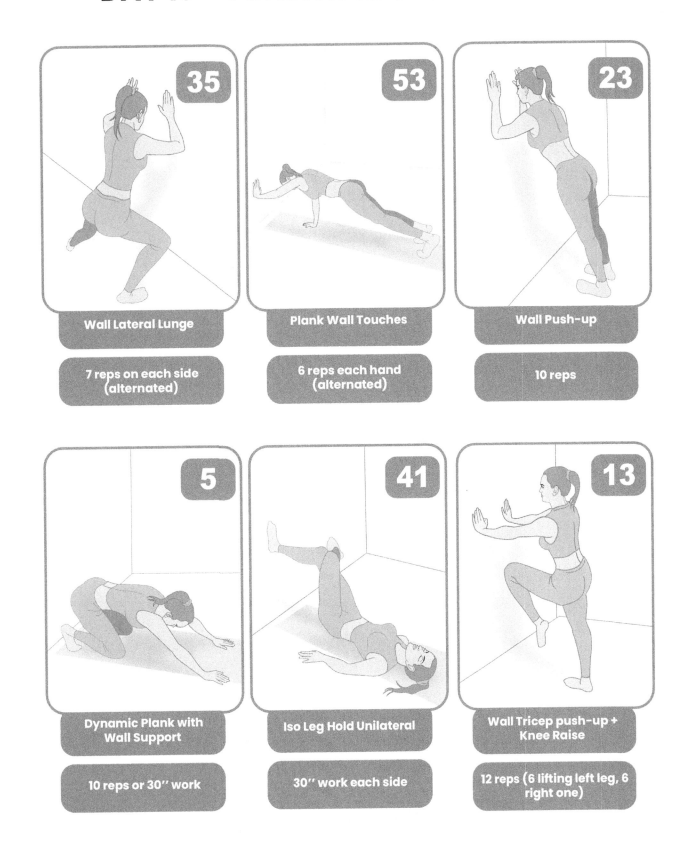

35 Wall Lateral Lunge
7 reps on each side (alternated)

53 Plank Wall Touches
6 reps each hand (alternated)

23 Wall Push-up
10 reps

5 Dynamic Plank with Wall Support
10 reps or 30'' work

41 Iso Leg Hold Unilateral
30'' work each side

13 Wall Tricep push-up + Knee Raise
12 reps (6 lifting left leg, 6 right one)

DAY 20 – Perform two to three sets

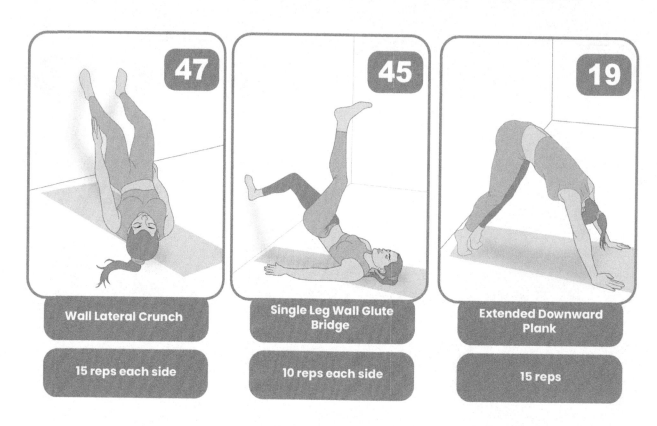

47

Wall Lateral Crunch

15 reps each side

45

Single Leg Wall Glute Bridge

10 reps each side

19

Extended Downward Plank

15 reps

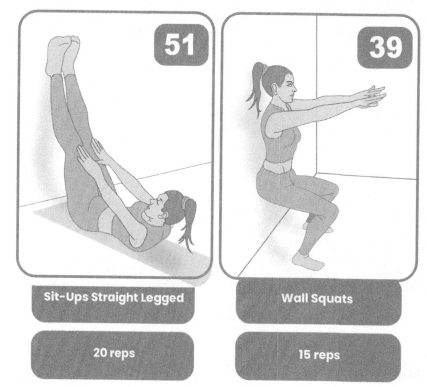

51

Sit-Ups Straight Legged

20 reps

39

Wall Squats

15 reps

DAY 21 – Perform three to four sets

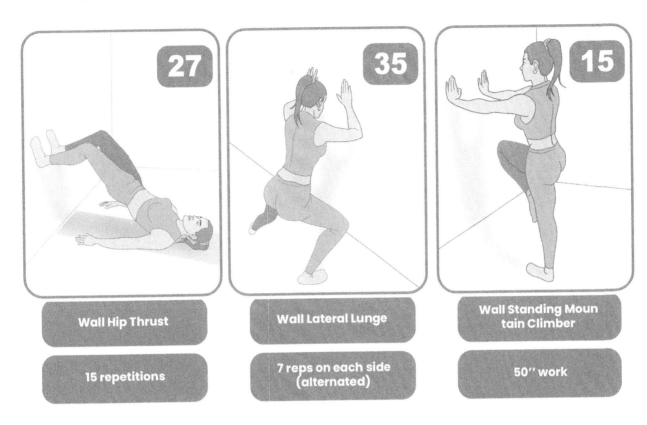

27

Wall Hip Thrust

15 repetitions

35

Wall Lateral Lunge

7 reps on each side (alternated)

15

Wall Standing Mountain Climber

50'' work

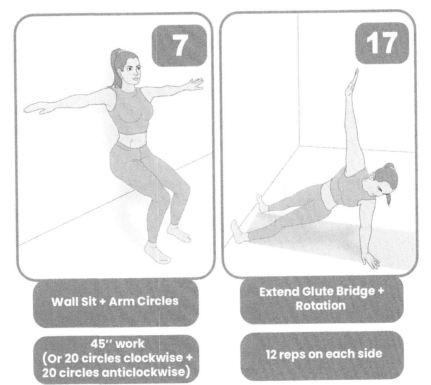

7

Wall Sit + Arm Circles

45'' work (Or 20 circles clockwise + 20 circles anticlockwise)

17

Extend Glute Bridge + Rotation

12 reps on each side

DAY 22 – Perform three to four sets

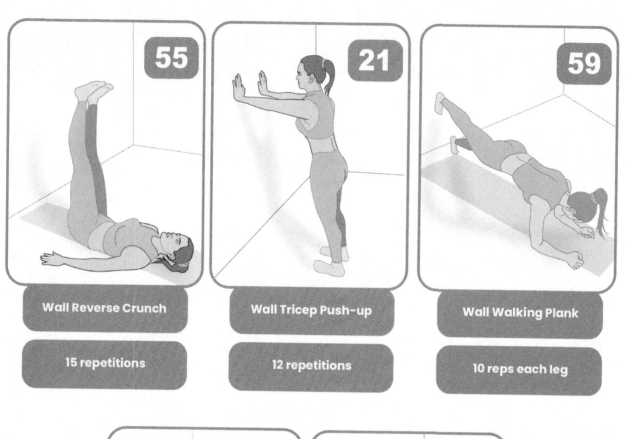

55

Wall Reverse Crunch

15 repetitions

21

Wall Tricep Push-up

12 repetitions

59

Wall Walking Plank

10 reps each leg

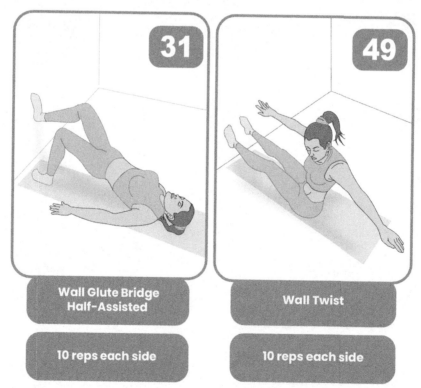

31

Wall Glute Bridge Half-Assisted

10 reps each side

49

Wall Twist

10 reps each side

DAY 23 – Perform three to four sets

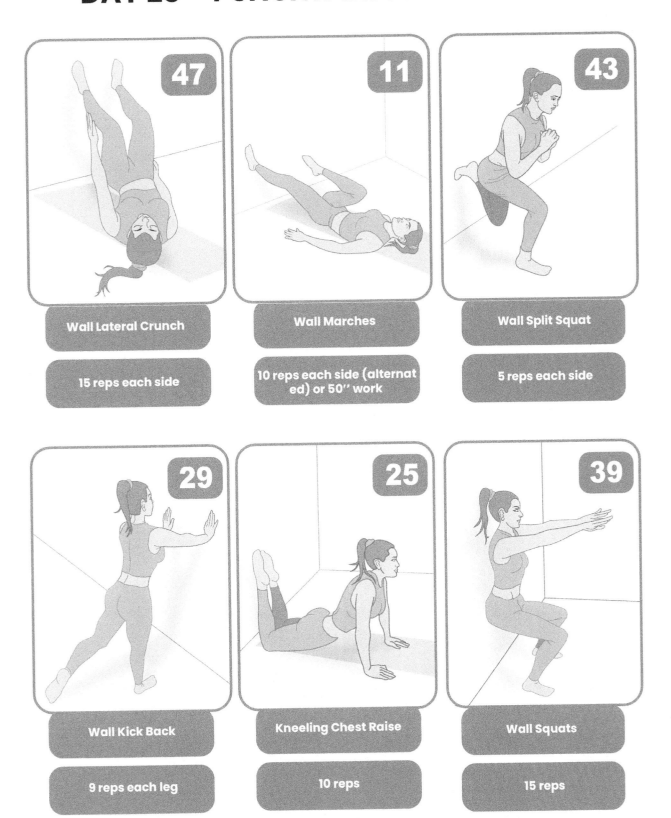

47 Wall Lateral Crunch
15 reps each side

11 Wall Marches
10 reps each side (alternated) or 50" work

43 Wall Split Squat
5 reps each side

29 Wall Kick Back
9 reps each leg

25 Kneeling Chest Raise
10 reps

39 Wall Squats
15 reps

DAY 24 – Perform three to four sets

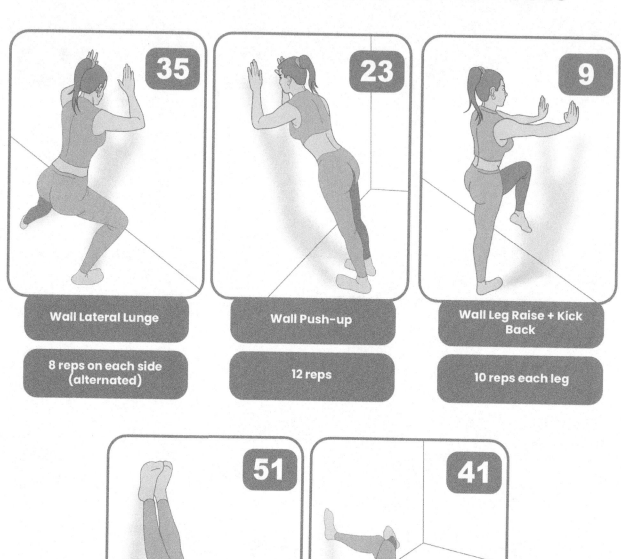

35
Wall Lateral Lunge
8 reps on each side (alternated)

23
Wall Push-up
12 reps

9
Wall Leg Raise + Kick Back
10 reps each leg

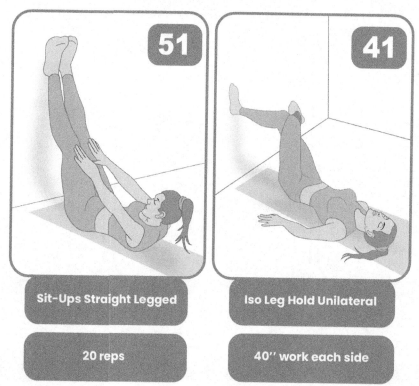

51
Sit-Ups Straight Legged
20 reps

41
Iso Leg Hold Unilateral
40'' work each side

DAY 25 – Perform three to four sets

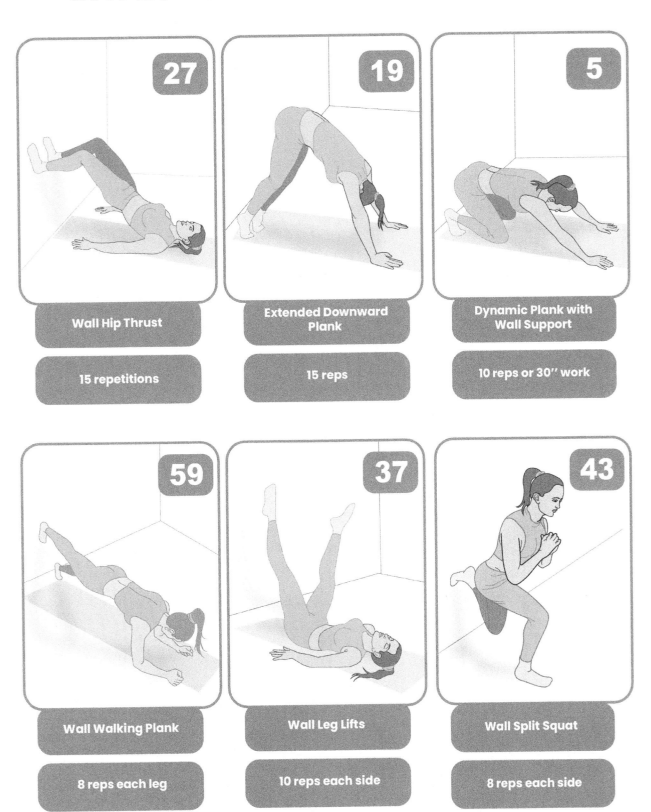

27	**19**	**5**
Wall Hip Thrust	Extended Downward Plank	Dynamic Plank with Wall Support
15 repetitions	15 reps	10 reps or 30" work
59	**37**	**43**
Wall Walking Plank	Wall Leg Lifts	Wall Split Squat
8 reps each leg	10 reps each side	8 reps each side

DAY 26 – Perform three to four sets

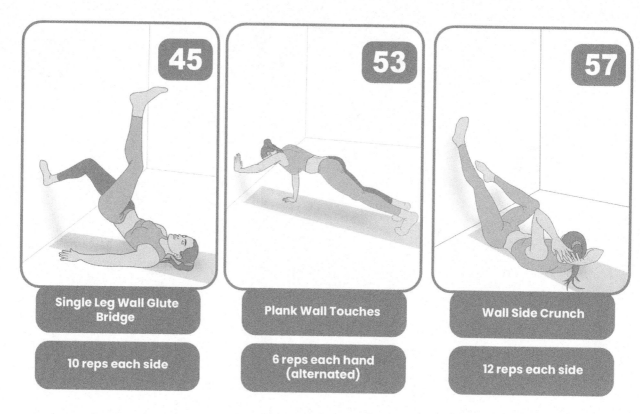

45

Single Leg Wall Glute Bridge

10 reps each side

53

Plank Wall Touches

6 reps each hand (alternated)

57

Wall Side Crunch

12 reps each side

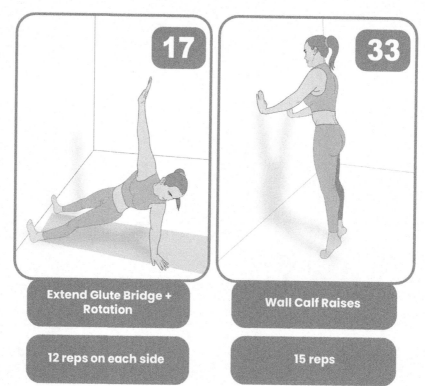

17

Extend Glute Bridge + Rotation

12 reps on each side

33

Wall Calf Raises

15 reps

DAY 27 – Perform three to four sets

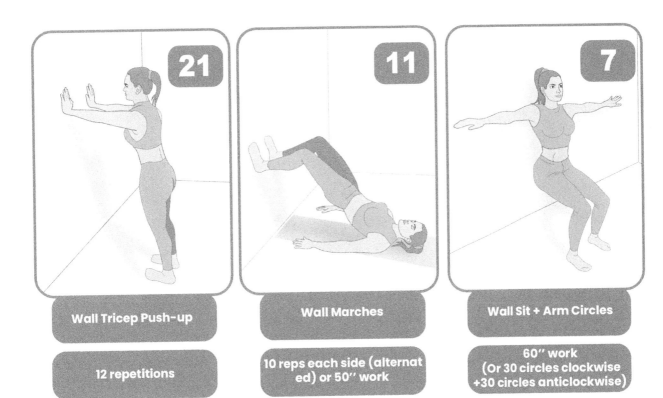

21

Wall Tricep Push-up

12 repetitions

11

Wall Marches

10 reps each side (alternated) or 50'' work

7

Wall Sit + Arm Circles

60'' work
(Or 30 circles clockwise
+30 circles anticlockwise)

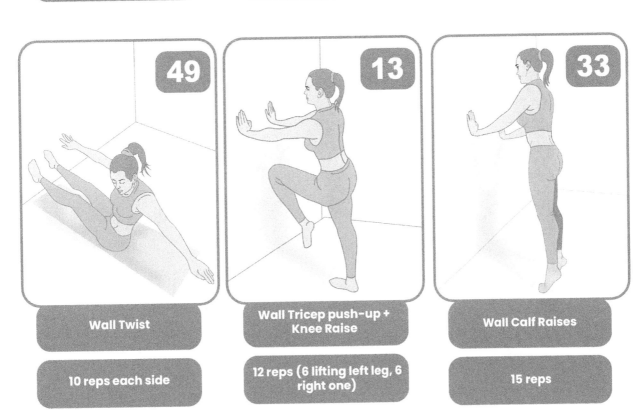

49

Wall Twist

10 reps each side

13

**Wall Tricep push-up +
Knee Raise**

12 reps (6 lifting left leg, 6
right one)

33

Wall Calf Raises

15 reps

DAY 28 – Perform three to four sets

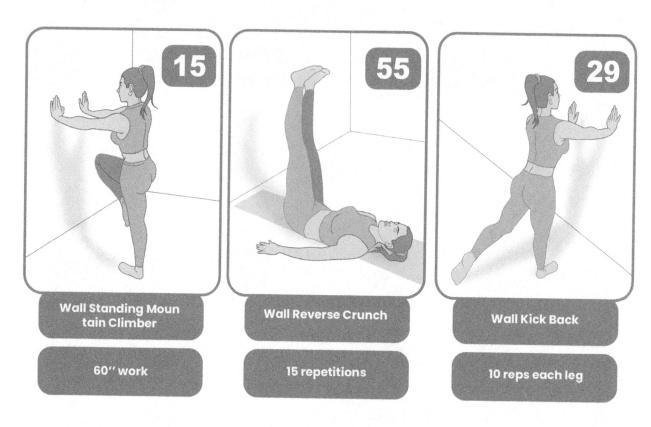

15

Wall Standing Moun tain Climber

60" work

55

Wall Reverse Crunch

15 repetitions

29

Wall Kick Back

10 reps each leg

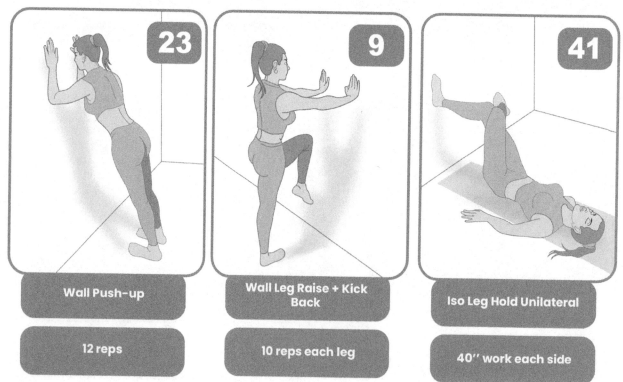

23

Wall Push-up

12 reps

9

Wall Leg Raise + Kick Back

10 reps each leg

41

Iso Leg Hold Unilateral

40" work each side

3 STRATEGIES TO TACKLE STRESS AND IMPROVE YOUR WELL-BEING.

As you know Wall Pilates exercises will give you lots of benefits. However, to live a stress-free life and feel at your best, exercise is not often enough. Your lifestyle and time the way you live is tremendously important. Therefore, I would like to recommend some guidelines to improve your health other than exercise! Those are applicable tips that will not cost any time extra and are simple life hacks that done consistently will be a game-changer!

● **Go outside in the morning and reduce blue lights.**

A morning walk outside has been shown to improve mood, focus, and well-being. Scientifically, this is why increase in cortisol early in the day which is good for our body. In fact, release in cortisol in large quantities happen roughly every 24 hours. By releasing it early in the morning, you will avoid a cortisol peak in the late afternoon or evening, making it difficult to fall asleep.

Many of the benefits of daily morning sunlight, ideally when there is the sunrise are:

▸ Mood and emotional control

▸ Sleep's quality improvement

▸ Regulations of hormones

▸ Improves focus and concentration

▸ Boost Immune system

Additionally, I would recommend reducing exposure to blue light drastically. Phones, laptops, and other devices are obviously needed during the day.

However, if after dinner or just the last hour before going to sleep, you implement the simple habit of taking some time off them, this will help you fall asleep faster and improve the quality of your sleep.

Lastly, bedtime and waking time are important. You will also be more vital during the day if you sleep at the same time every day. There were some people I used to train in London that a few hours of sleep less or more would make all the difference in terms of energy during the session as well as overall mood. I am sure you can relate!

● Eat considerably and stay away from alcohol and caffeine.

Not only quality but also quantity is important. Many people, once they start focusing on their fitness, switch from junk food to healthier food to get fit and lose weight. However, they end up eating more calories than before.

Eating quality food does not mean that you can eat them regardless of the amount of it. Be considerate.

A tip that can help you increase satiety is to drink more water, especially before meals. As well as starting your meals with fruit and vegetables. However, for more accurate information on diet and nutrition consult a specialist.

Also, alcohol consumption is something that does not benefit you neither for physical health nor for mental health. In the long run, even a small amount of alcohol consumed daily/weekly can lead to a decrease in resilience and stress. You should avoid this if you want to level up!

Caffeine is also not a great thing to take daily. If you are used to it, keep drinking your coffee. However, I would not take it the first 90 minutes after waking up. Andrew Hubermann, a well-known researcher, studied the effects of caffeine intake in the morning. It seems to be leading to a crash in energy in the early afternoon. Waiting just 90' after waking to drink a cup of coffee seems not to create this effect.

This is something you might want to try!

- **Take 10 min a day for "Breath".**

This is an exercise that can be done anywhere without any cost. Do it for a week and you will be more centered, calm in stressful situations and your sleep is going to improve as well.

Personally, I recommend using NSDR from any YouTube video. It is a guided meditation that I personally find helpful and effective for improving my sleep, ability to stay calm in stressful situations as well as improving my mood. Also, it is easier to do than meditating, especially for beginners.

CONCLUSION

Here you have everything you need to tone up and feel better about yourself by simply training at home with only a wall! Wall Pilates can really give you lots of benefits, making your waist slimmer, being more flexible and overall healthier.

The reason why wall Pilates works like magic is that:

- it does not necessarily feel like an excruciating workout. Most people are not consistent with exercise because at times exercise selection is too difficult and it feels overwhelming. Wall Pilates is doable but challenging.

I am a strong believer that you should end a workout feeling better than how you started it! Yes, feeling tired at times is normal but if every time you end a training you are exhausted, you are destroying your body rather than making it stronger and fitter. Wall Pilates is the perfect combination making the workout challenging enough as well as not too intense.

- Secondly, these exercises are fun! None of my clients, both online and offline, ever gave me negative feedback on these exercises. They can be adjustable to any fitness level to make it challenging enough, and you move your body in ways that it feels like you are exploring a new part of yourself rather than doing very static movements.

- Thirdly, being home exercises, there is no excuse for not having time to commute to the gym or not having the right equipment. Either in the morning, lunch break or evening time, take 10-20' for yourself and change your life once and for all!

With Wall Pilates Workout for Women and the 28-Day Plan you are having the blueprint to reshape your body, tone your abs and have a slim waist!

ABOUT ME

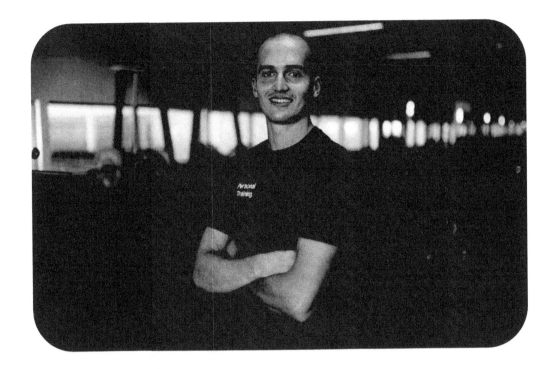

My name is Alessandro, I am Italian, and I have lived in Milan, London, and Valencia, Spain. My passion for fitness started in my childhood and never stopped since then.

I am a certified Personal Trainer with years of experience in the United Kingdom and Spain. I have been studying fitness articles and guides to make people fitter for years. My experience helping hundreds of people led me to write numerous books on it.

The goal is to make them healthier, more flexible, stronger, and enjoy life more. I have been doing 1-on-1 sessions, group sessions, and online coaching with people of all ages.

I dream of a world in which age is just a number in which everyone is fit regardless of their schedule...with just 10 minutes per day and a good lifestyle people underestimate the results they can get, and this is the message I love to spread across with the books I have been publishing.

Unlock 14 days of personalized coaching, Relaxation Breathing Techniques, and a nutrition guide. Ready to transform? ⭐

➡️📱 SCAN NOW and amplify your results! 🌈

It's not over yet, there's another surprise for you.
Book now for your free 1-on-1 Wall Pilates session with me! Simply write 'FREE CALL' to avfitness99coaching@gmail.com, and let's schedule a training together

💪 Other Books Available for you on Amazon 💪

1. **Wall Pilates for Seniors: Rediscover The Joy of Movement and Become Independent Once Again with Low-Impact Exercises to Improve Flexibility and Balance**

   Fantastic to approach Wall Pilates exercises with low-impact exercises in just 10-15 minutes per day - Plan of 30 days included.

2. **Wall Pilates Workouts: 28-Day Challenge with Exercise Chart for Weight Loss | 10-Min Routines for Women, Beginners and Seniors - Color Illustrated Edition**

   The newest book! Fully colored, Video tutorials, graphic routines and downloadable exercise charts ... .the best to lose weight and burn fat at home!

3. **Chair Exercises for Seniors: Rediscover Pain-Free Daily Activities with A Step-by-Step Illustrated Workout to Improve Balance and Strength in Just 10 Minutes a Day**

   Plenty of exercises and fantastic routines to stay fit and get more flexible with easy-to-follow exercises!

4. **Chair Yoga for Seniors: 28-Day Challenge for Weight Loss with Exercise Chart | 10-Min Low-Impact Routines for Beginners - Color Illustrated Edition**

   Color illustrated, easy-to-follow, step-by-step illustrations, printable exercise charts and direct access to text me anytime you need...

5. **Chair Yoga for Weight Loss: 28-Day Challenge to Lose Belly Fat Sitting Down with Low-Impact Exercises in Just 10 Minutes Per Day**

   Arguably the best book to burn calories, lose weight and improve flexibility

6. Balance Exercises Bible for Seniors: 12-Week Plan to Prevent Falls and Walking with Confidence in Under 10 Minutes a Day | Pictures Included for Easy Understanding

Plenty of exercises to choose from for beginners, intermediate and advanced - 12-week plan and so much more!

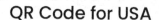 Scan the QR Code to Go to My Amazon Profile and Get the Book you Prefer 👇

QR Code for USA

QR Code for UK

QR Code for Canada

Fo any questions or doubts email me at avfitness99coaching@gmail.com

Made in the USA
Columbia, SC
29 October 2024

45239418R00063